## Other Books by Bill Reynolds

Bodybuilding for Beginners

Boyer and Valerie Coe's Weight Training Book (with Boyer and Valerie Coe)

Complete Weight Training Book

Flex Appeal by Rachel (with Rachel McLish)

Getting Built! (with Dr. Lynne Pirie)

The Gold's Gym Book of Bodybuilding (with Ken Sprague)

The Gold's Gym Nutrition Bible (with Peter Grymkowski  et al.)

The Gold's Gym Training Encyclopedia (with Peter Grymkowski  et al.)

Joe Weider's Bodybuilding Encyclopedia (with Joe Weider)

Mr. Olympia's Muscle Mastery (with Samir Bannout)

Peak Physique (with Albert Beckles)

Pro-Style Bodybuilding (with Tom Platz)

Solid Gold (with Peter Grymkowski  et al.)

Supercut (with Joyce L. Vedral, Ph.D.)

The Weider System of Bodybuilding (with Joe Weider)

Weight Training for Beginners

Winning Women's Bodybuilding (with Laura Combes)

# Freestyle
# BODYBUILDING

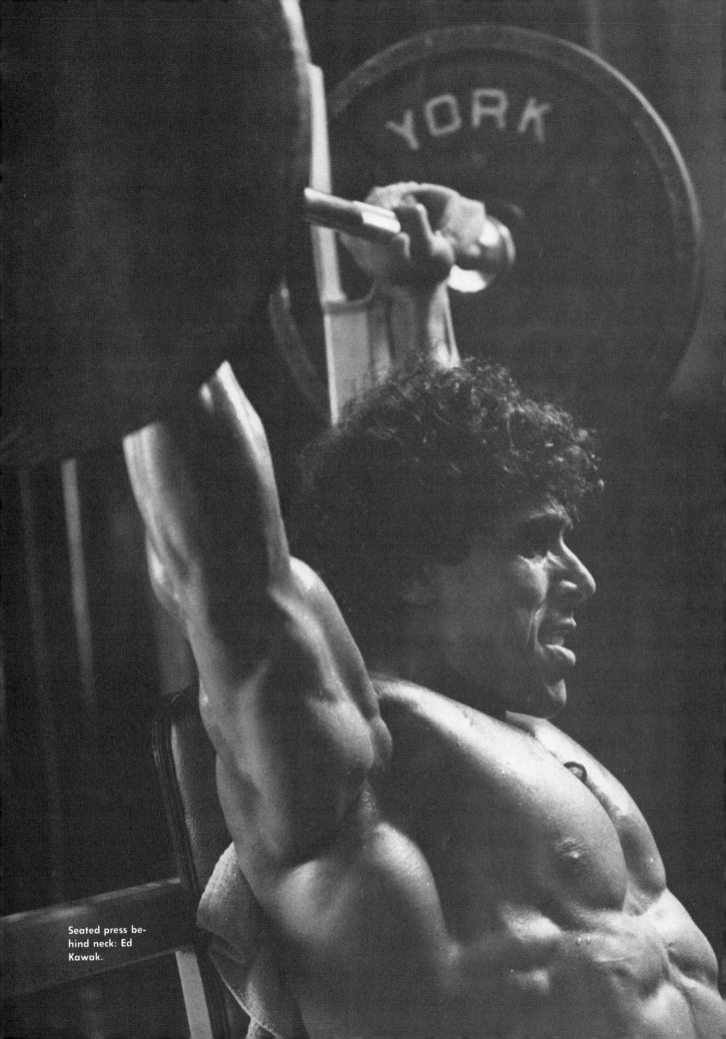

Seated press behind neck: Ed Kawak.

# Freestyle
# BODYBUILDING

## Bill Reynolds

EDITOR IN CHIEF, FLEX

## Chris Lund

PHOTOGRAPHY

A Perigee Book

Perigee Books
are published by
The Putnam Publishing Group
200 Madison Avenue
New York, NY 10016

Photographs by Chris Lund

Library of Congress Cataloging-in-Publication Data

Reynolds, Bill.
    Freestyle bodybuilding / by Bill Reynolds; photography by Chris Lund.
    p. cm.
    "A Perigee book."
    ISBN 0-399-51453-8: Price
    1. Bodybuilding.    I. Lund, Chris.    II. Title.
GV546. 5R484 1988
646.7'5—dc19                    88-9774 CIP

Design by The Sarabande Press
Printed in the United States of America
1   2   3   4   5   6   7   8   9   10

*To Sho Fukushima, my friend
and former graduate school office mate,
who opened my mind to Oriental thought.*

# Contents

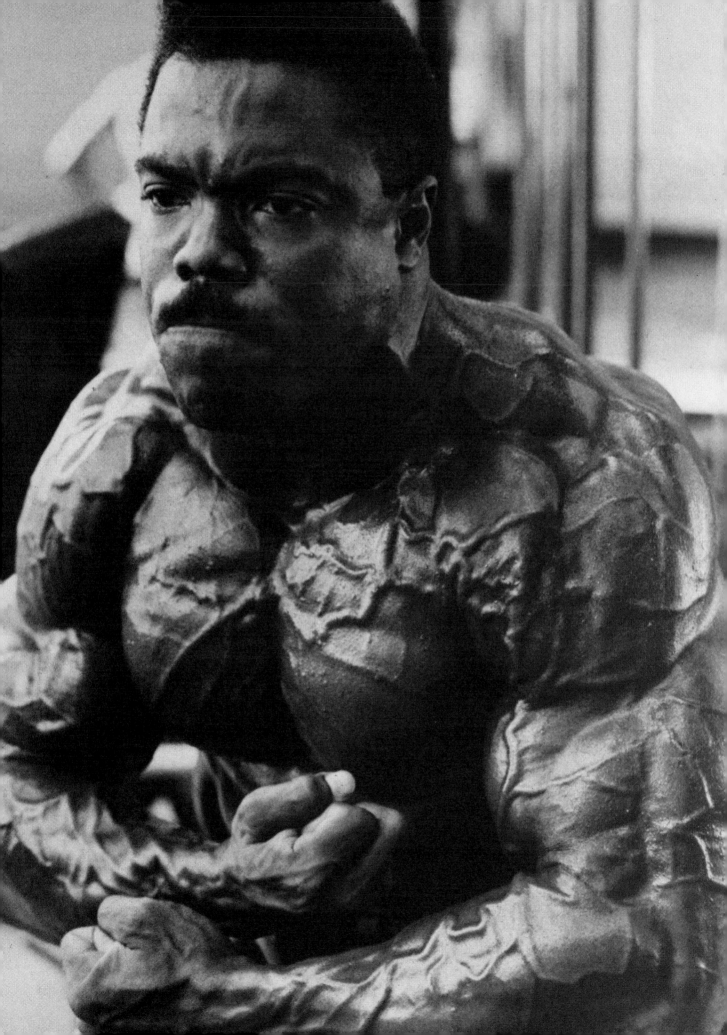

# 1

# The Mind and Bodybuilding

**T**he mind is your biggest muscle," says four-time Mr. Olympia Lee Haney. "In general, bodybuilding is fifty-fifty training and nutrition, but the world's most perfect diet and all of the training in the world won't build an ounce of muscle mass if your mind isn't totally into the bodybuilding process.

"I began training fifteen years ago, and gradually mastered the mental aspect of the sport. The more I learned about the mind and bodybuilding, the more convinced I became that it was the single most important factor in building huge, high-quality muscles. Without having trained my mind to build big muscles, I would never have won the major titles which have come my way over the years."

When I first became aware of the importance of my mind in building muscles, I was a 27-year-old competitor visiting the legendary Gold's Gym in Venice, California, for the first time. I'd driven my aged Volkswagen more than 1000 miles down from Seattle to meet Arnold Schwarzenegger, Frank Zane, Franco Columbu, Ken Waller and all of the other IFBB champions who were training there at the time.

◄ The absolutely incredible Phil Hill.

I waited patiently for Arnold Schwarzenegger, the reigning Mr. Olympia at the time, to finish his workout. After he showered, I tremulously asked him if he'd tell me the secret to his success. "It's all in the mind," he answered. "I'm the best bodybuilder in the sport because my mind is stronger and better disciplined than others'. I know what I want and I go after it.

"One of my mental secrets is that I always think big. Ever since I was a boy, I've had these fantastic visions of what I wanted to one day become. These were daydreams that just popped into my mind, not something I

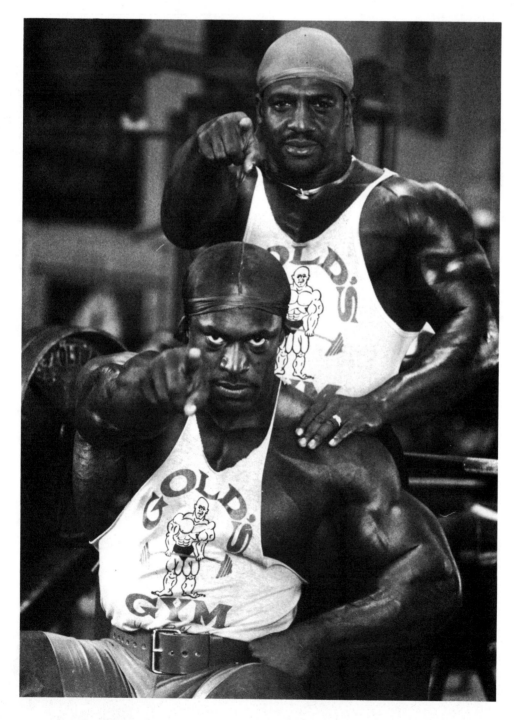

◄ "Look out! We're a'coming," declare Lee Haney and Superman Blount.

Heavy T-bar rows ➤ are great for back thickness. Gary Strydom uses them here.

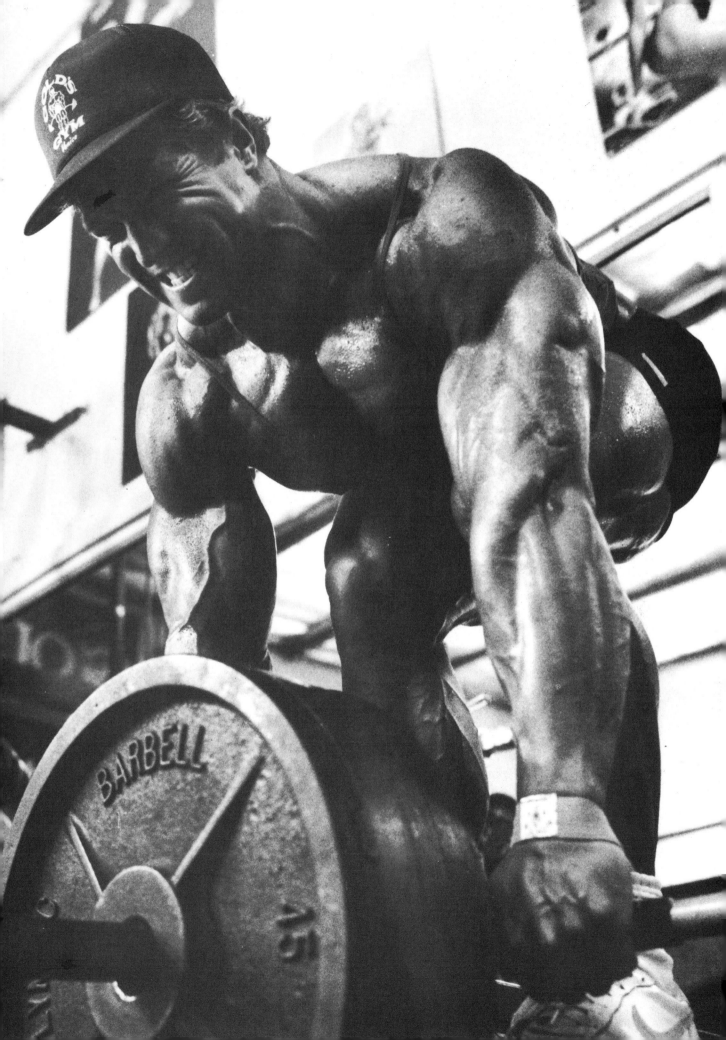

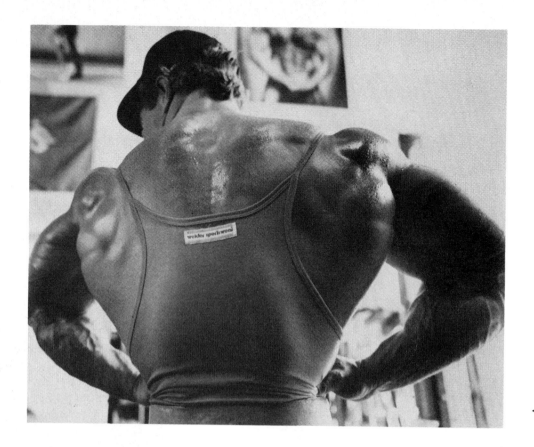

consciously planned. But I gradually grew to believe that I would definitely become the greatest bodybuilder in the sport.

"I also think big when it comes to visualizing my physique the way I wanted it to be. When I was working my biceps, I imagined them being as big as the Matterhorn. And that got me over the problem of having a barrier to my arm measurement. Most bodybuilders start thinking about having an 18-inch arm measurement, and they never seem to achieve that level of development. It becomes a barrier for them. But when I think of my biceps as being as huge as a mountain in the Alps, there is no barrier."

Arnold had a point, because he had the largest and most muscular arms of any bodybuilder currently competing. I began to learn the process of mental visualization, using it in my workouts. Within a few months I won my first title, and continued to win quite regularly until I had reached my goals in bodybuilding. Then I stepped out of competition.

As I began to write magazine articles on bodybuilding, I learned more and more about the mental aspect of the sport. The more I learned, the more convinced I became that this was the key ingredient in the success formula of every champion bodybuilder.

I heard different pieces of mental training knowledge from most of the bodybuilders I interviewed, and particularly from Frank Zane (three times Mr. Olympia and a legend in the sport), Tom Platz (Mr. Universe) and Sue Ann McKean (California Champion and a leading pro bodybuilder).

Phil Hill. ➤

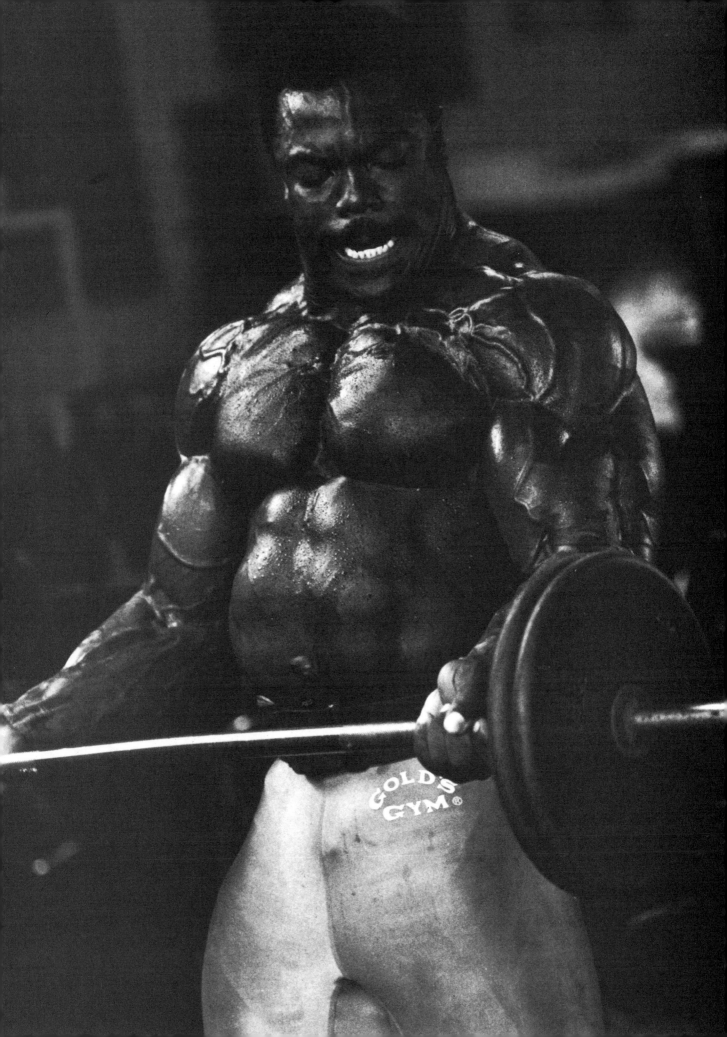

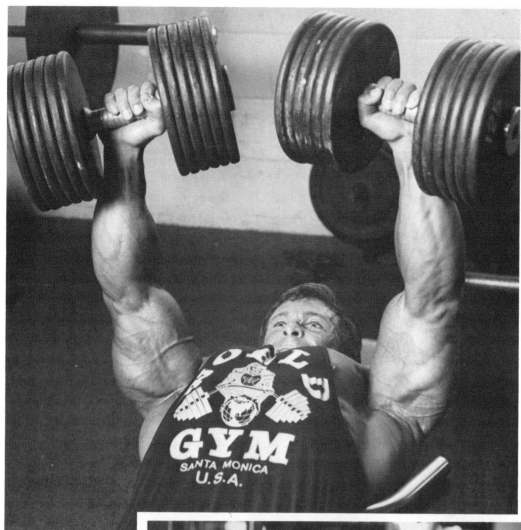

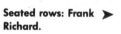

Seated rows: Frank ➤
Richard.

◄ Very heavy dumb-
bell bench presses
are another great
chest builder:
Graeme Lancefield.

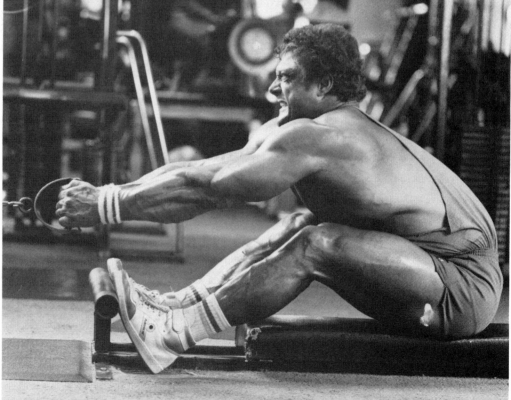

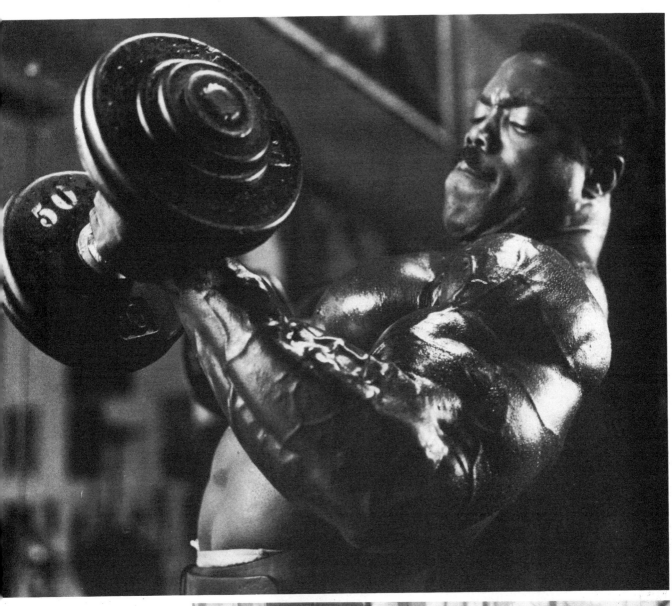

▲ The incredible Phil Hill.

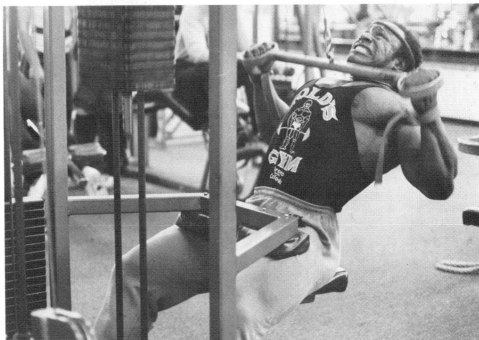

Parallel grip pull-downs place the biceps in a much stronger position: Lee Haney. ▶

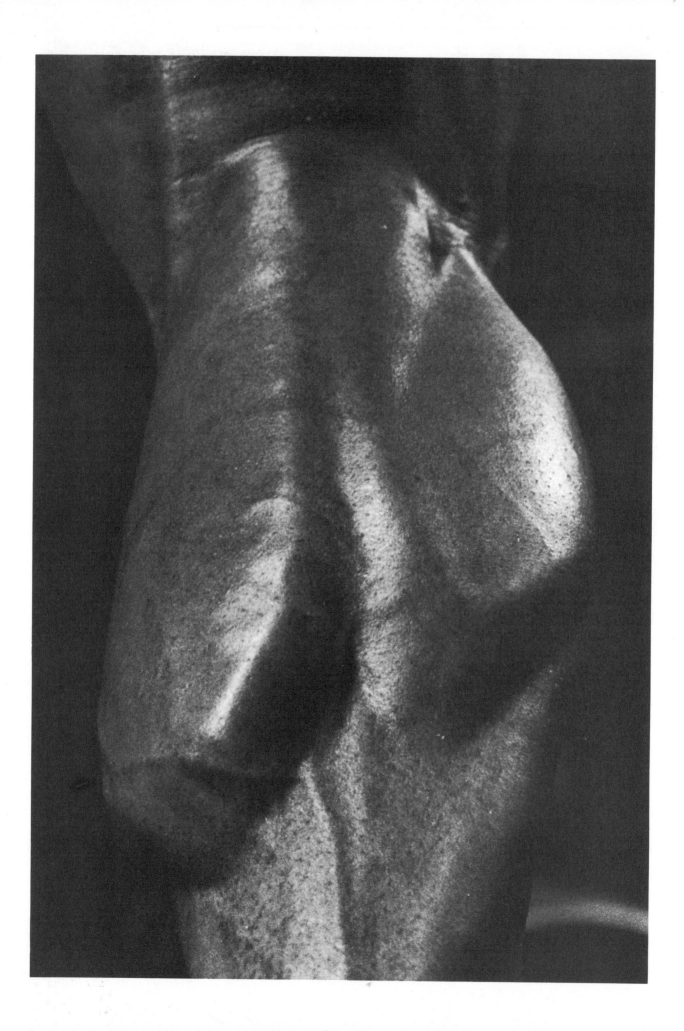

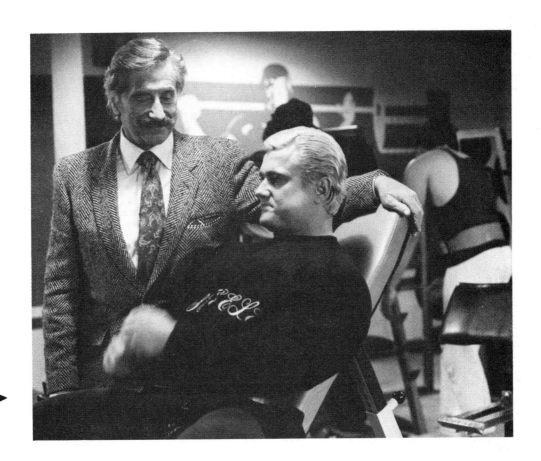

Joe Weider (standing) and Tom Platz on the set of the movie *Flex*.

Over a period of years I concluded that every aspect of the bodybuilding mental approach—as covered in this book—could be represented by the Zen Buddhist way of approaching life. As Zen Master Rama (Dr. Frederick Lenz) writes, "Zen Buddhist thought has had a profound influence upon Chinese and Japanese history and culture. A great deal of the current success of the Japanese corporate mind stems from the effect of centuries of Zen practice in Japan. Martial arts, dance, poetry, the tea ceremony and many other forms of personal, athletic and artistic expression have been given birth to by Zen mind.

"Zen is a highly refined and artistic approach to the meaning of life. It isn't necessary to learn Oriental customs or to speak the Japanese language to successfully practice it. All that is required is an open mind, patience, a good sense of humor and an intense desire for self-improvement."

Daisetz T. Suzuki has written numerous books and monographs on Zen Buddhism. In his *Zen and Japanese Culture* he proposes the following eleven elements as a summary of Zen:

- Zen discipline consists in attaining enlightenment (or *satori,* in Japanese).
- *Satori* finds a meaning hitherto hidden in our daily concrete particular experiences, such as eating, drinking, or business of all kinds.

◄ Gary Strydom's calf.

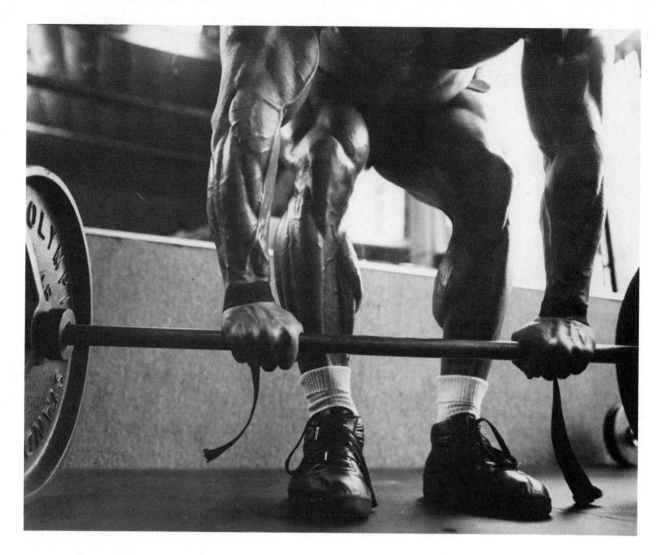

A Scott Wilson.

- The meaning thus revealed is not something added from the outside. It is in being itself, in becoming itself, in living itself. This is called, in Japanese, a life of *kono-mama* or *sono-mama*. *Kono-* or *sono-mama* means the "isness" of a thing. Reality is its isness.
- Some may say, "There cannot be any meaning in mere isness." But this is not the view held by Zen, for according to it, isness is the meaning. When I see into it I see it as clearly as I see myself reflected in a mirror.
- This is what made Ho Kōji (P'ang Chü-shih) a lay disciple of the eighth century, declare:

> How wondrous this, how mysterious!
> I carry fuel, I draw water.

The fuel carrying or the water drawing itself, apart from its utilitarianism, is full of meaning; hence its "wonder," its "mystery."

A close-up of Scott Wilson's superb calves.

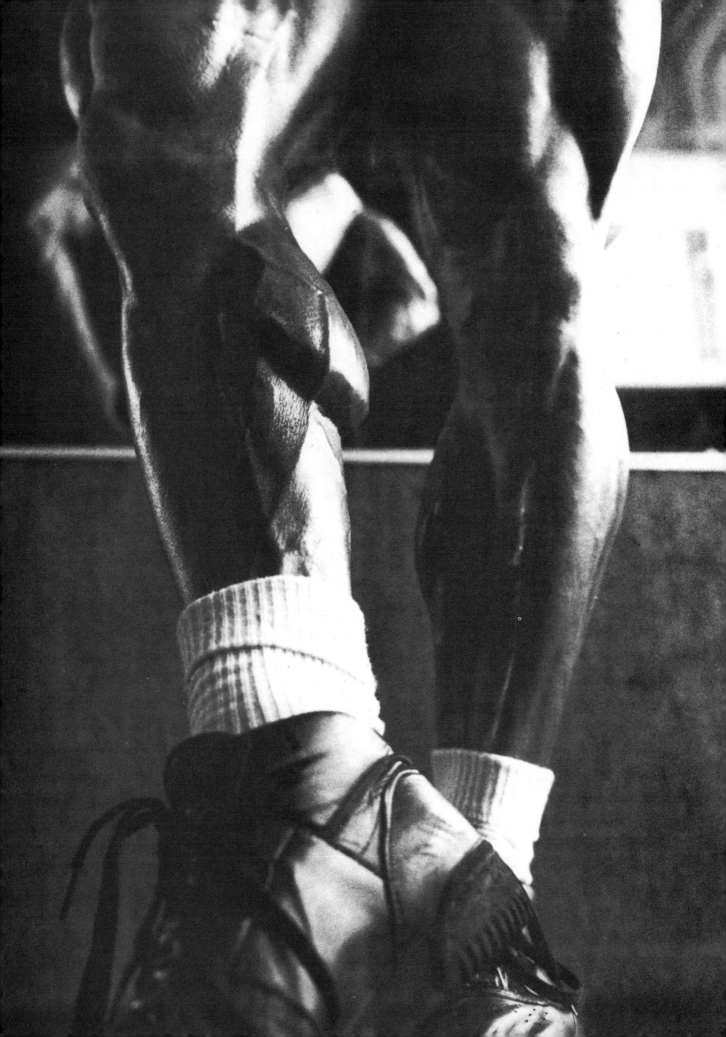

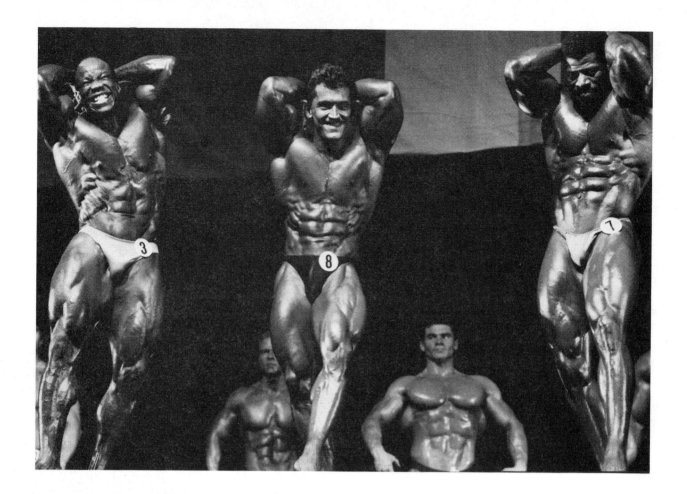

- Zen does not, therefore, indulge in abstraction or in conceptualization. In its verbalism it may sometimes appear that Zen does this a great deal. But this is an error most commonly entertained by those who do not at all know Zen.
- *Satori* is emancipation, moral, spiritual, as well as intellectual. When I am in my isness, thoroughly purged of all intellectual sediments, I have my freedom in its primary sense.
- When the mind, now abiding in its isness—which, to use Zen verbalism, is no isness—and thus free from intellectual complexities and moralistic attachments of every description, surveys the world of the senses in all its multiplicities, it discovers in it all sorts of values hitherto hidden from sight. Here opens to the artist a world full of wonders and miracles.
- The artist's world is one of free creation, and this can come only from intuitions directly and immediately rising from the isness of things, unhampered by senses and intellect. He creates forms and sounds out of formlessness and soundlessness. To this extent, the artist's world coincides with that of Zen.
- What differentiates Zen from the arts is this: While artists have

▲ Left to right: Al Beckles, Lee Labrada and Ron Love.

Lee Haney clinches ➤ yet another Mr. Olympia title.

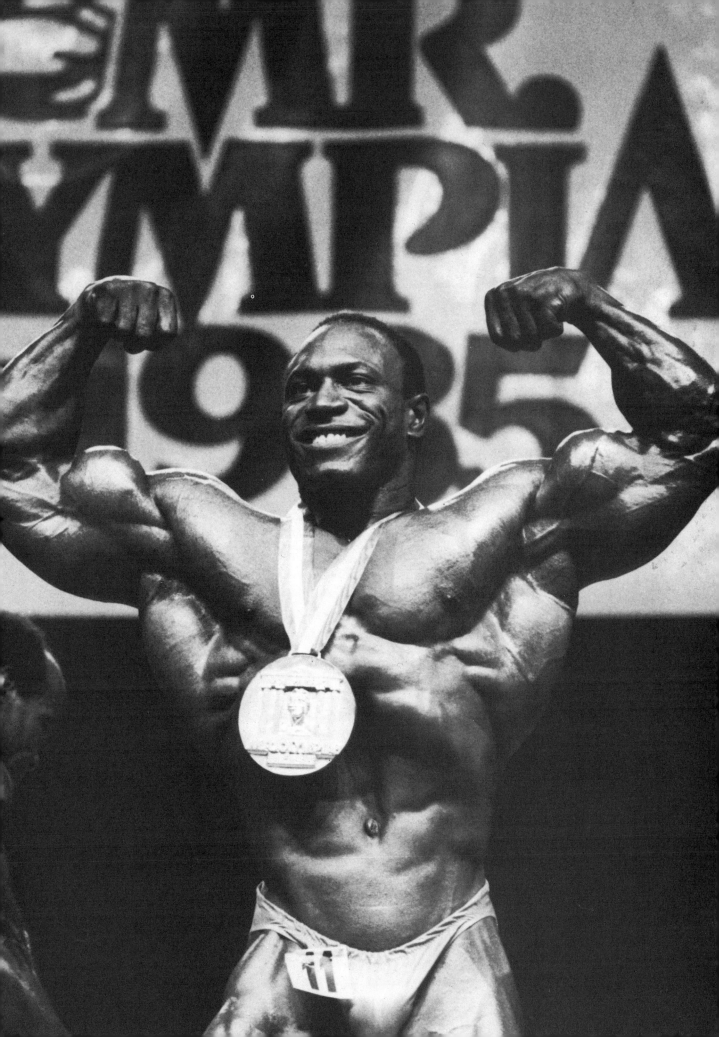

to resort to canvas and brush or mechanical instruments or some other medium to express themselves, Zen has no need of things external, except "the body" in which the Zen-man is, so to speak, embodied. From the absolute point of view this is not quite correct; I say it only in concession to the worldly way of saying things. What Zen does is to delineate itself on the infinite canvas of time and space the way the flying wild geese cast their shadow on the water below without any idea of doing so, while the water reflects the geese just as naturally and unintentionally.

• The Zen-man is an artist to the extent that, as the sculptor chisels out a great figure deeply buried in a mass of inert matter, the Zen-man transforms his own life into a work of creation, which exists, as Christians might say, in the mind of God.

This is only a brief summary of Zen, a starting point for you in your deeper study of the mental aspect of bodybuilding. I have listed several excellent books on Zen in the reading list at the end of this book. I particularly recommend Suzuki's texts.

Left to right: Mike Christian, Rich Gaspari, and Roy Callendar.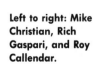

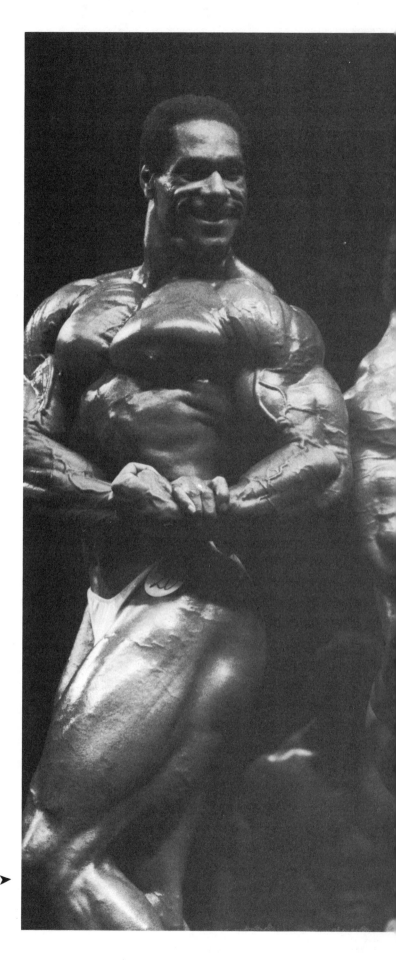

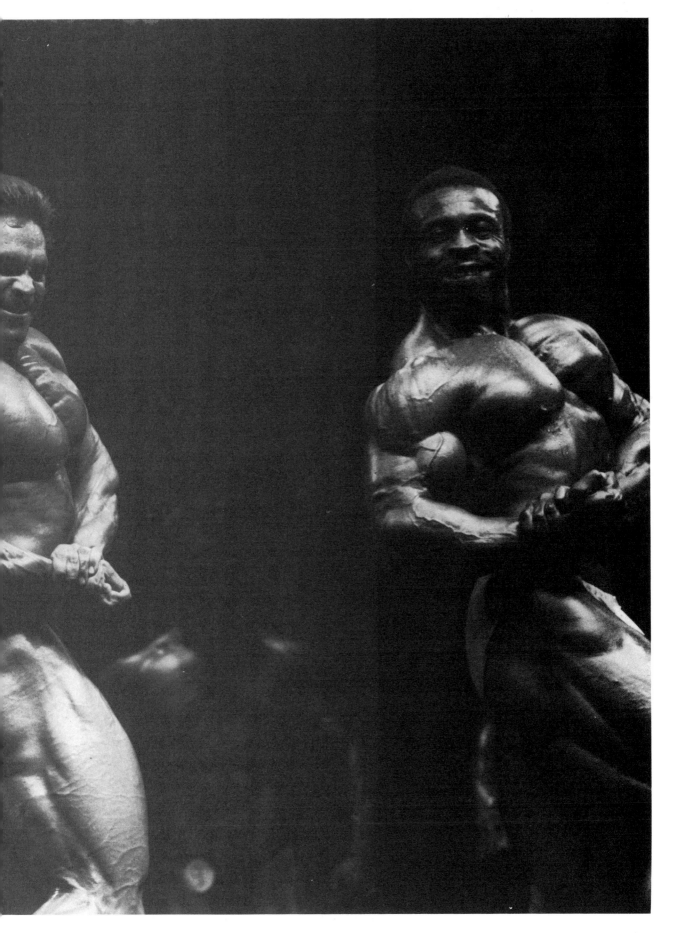

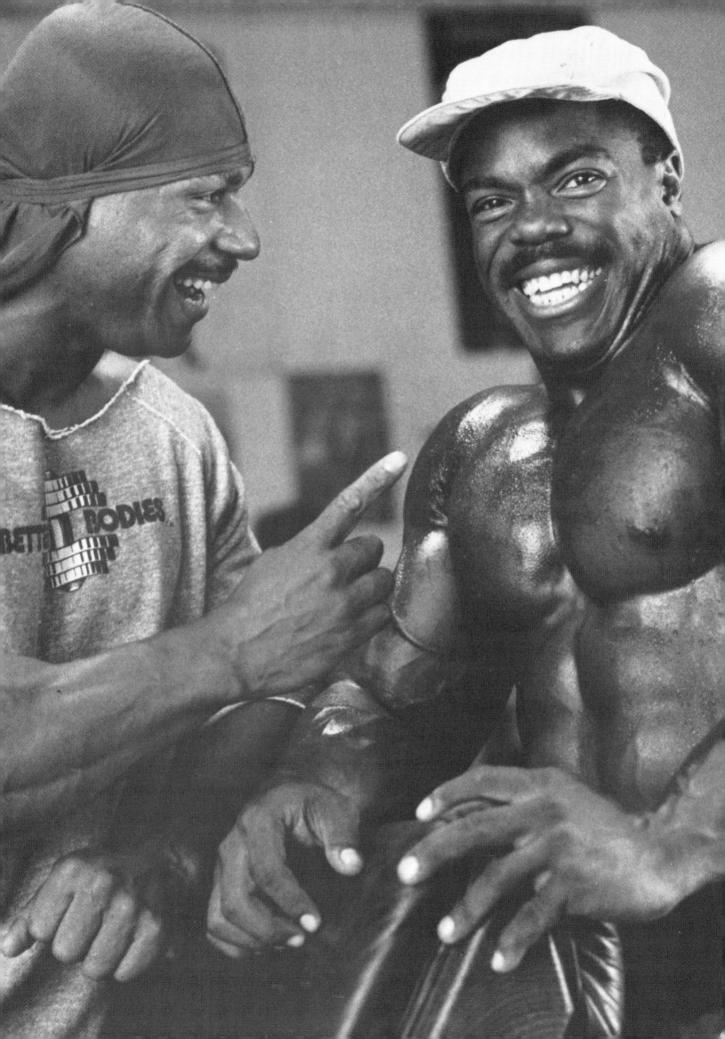

# 2

# Goal Setting

The essence of goal setting in bodybuilding and other activities has been set forth in this aphorism from Lao-tzu, founder of Taoism: "The journey of a thousand miles is started with a single step."

In this chapter I will explain this concept, that a distant goal can be reached by taking one step, then another and another, ad infinitum, until the goal stands before you. Bodybuilding is the most brutal sport on earth—particularly when you are forced to train with your normal high degree of intensity while concurrently following an energy-depleting precontest diet—and you'll need all of the help you can get in order to succeed at it. Proper use of goal setting will be enormously helpful in bringing you success as a competitive bodybuilder.

In order to get the most out of your efforts in bodybuilding, you must have a road map that shows the direct route to your goal. This is where the concept of a journey comes into practice. Your road map—a written sequential series of goals—puts you on a superhighway to success and keeps you from wasting time going down unproductive dead-end alleys.

In the same way you would take step after step along a journey, reaching

◄ Mike Christian jokes with big Phil Hill at Gold's Gym, California.

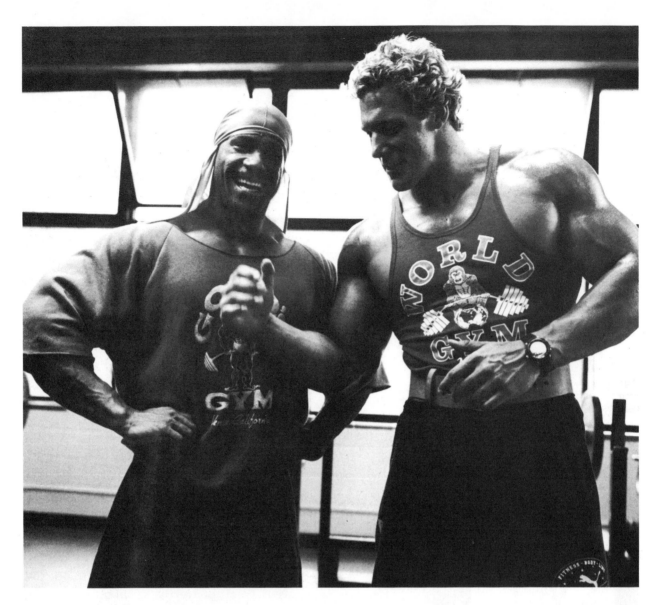

Mike Christian and ▲
Ralf Moeller joking
around at World
Gym.

an inn where you can rest each night, you do all of the sets and reps of a particular workout each day. And in the same way you plod from one inn to another until you reach the end of your journey, you continue to do workout after workout until you reach your goal in the sport, winning a particular bodybuilding title.

Each bodybuilder should set three types of goals. One of these, the supreme goal, never changes, but the other two lesser types of goals are constantly upgraded each time one is reached successfully.

Goals make your long journey in the sport of bodybuilding much easier to accept mentally. Few men can truly conceptualize walking a thousand miles or winning the Mr. Olympia title (Ms. Olympia for women). Both are truly mind-boggling goals. However, it is much easier to mentally accept a walk of ten miles or the gain of one pound of solid muscle tissue. If you take enough ten-mile strolls, you'll eventually walk a thousand miles. And if you make enough one-pound gains in muscular body weight, you might eventually become a Pro World Champion or Mr./Ms. Olympia. You need only to take that single step, followed by thousands and thousands of additional steps, and you will reach your goal.

### The Supreme Goal

As I mentioned, you should establish three types of goals in bodybuilding. The first and highest should be your supreme goal, the highest title to which you can aspire. There can be no other supreme goal except winning the Mr. or Ms. Olympia title.

If you are a serious bodybuilder, all of your efforts must be directed toward winning the Olympia. Chances are very slim indeed that you *will* win the Olympia—only eight men have won Mr. Olympia and only four women have taken the Ms. Olympia title—but you must still aspire to one day wear the Mr. or Ms. Olympia crown. And you have to want to reach that goal more than you have ever wanted anything else. This desire will ultimately fuel a burning quest to win all of the smaller titles leading up to a World Championship, which qualifies all bodybuilders for the Olympia, then to win the Olympia itself.

▼ High-intensity preacher curls with Ralf Moeller.

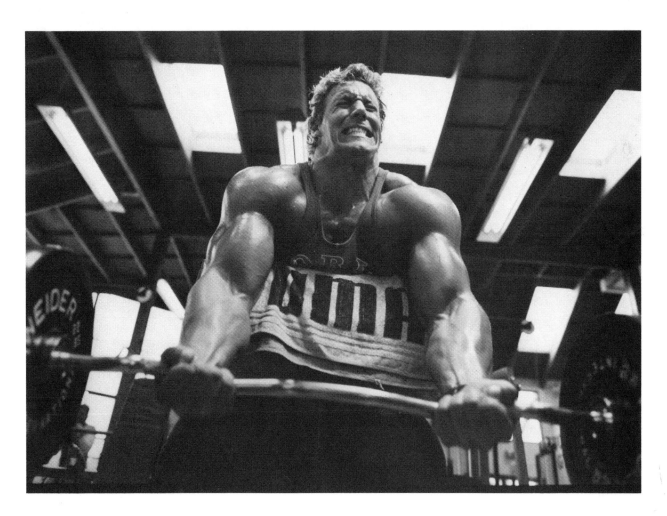

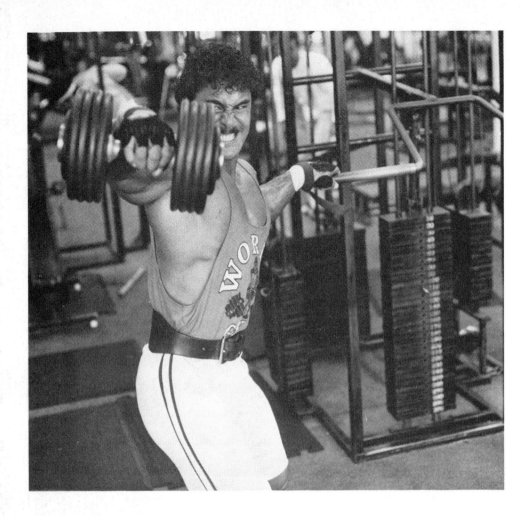

◄ Jon Aranita uses incredible poundages on all his shoulder movements. Here he does one-arm side laterals.

## Long-range Goals

The second type of goal you should set, which you will probably revise each year, is called a long-term goal. Most frequently, long-range goals are set in terms of a title that should be won during that year, with each year's title set successively higher than the one the previous year.

Four-time Mr. Olympia—and quite possibly the greatest bodybuilder in the history of the sport—Lee Haney tells how he set his own long-term goals over the years: "My first long-term bodybuilding goal was to win a regional-level teenage contest, then later the Teenage National Championship. Even though I knew very little about training and diet at the time—nor much about goal setting for that matter—I was successful in both quests. I not only won the Teenage Coastal USA Championship, but also the open Coastal USA Championship the same evening. And I climaxed my year by winning the Teen Nationals.

"My goal for the next year was to win a national title, specifically the Junior National Championship. But no matter how completely you plan sometimes, fate steps in and ruins all of those plans. In this case, I seriously injured my wrist, which ultimately required surgery and a lengthy period

Dave Hawk does ➤ alternate dumbbell curls.

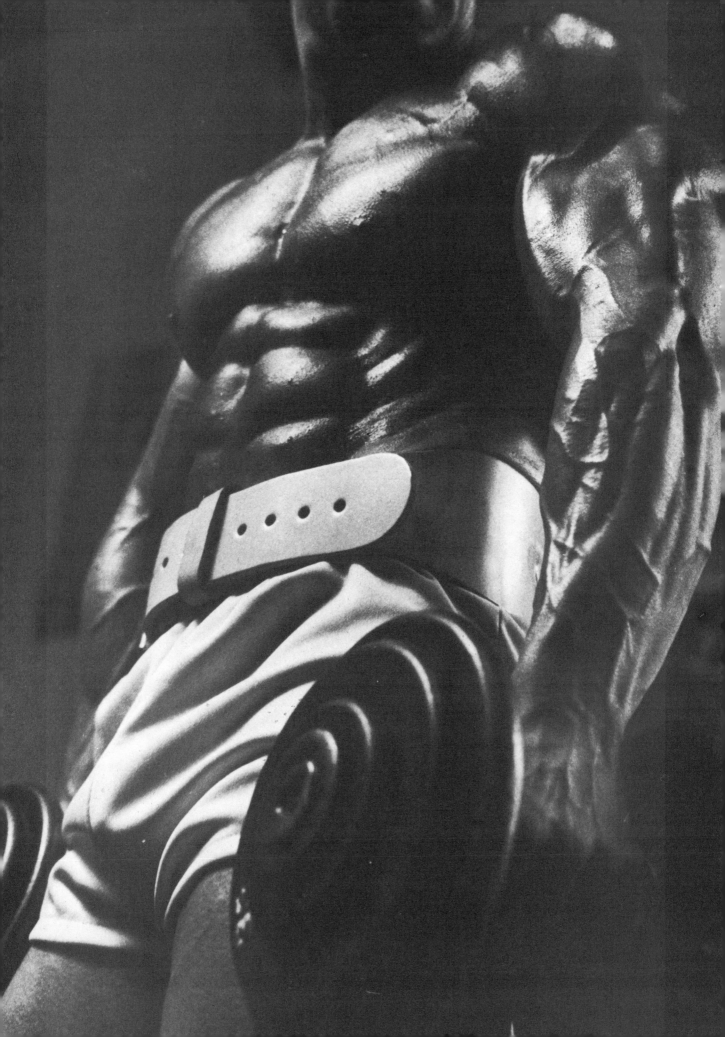

of rehabilitation. That injury blew an entire year's plans right out of the window.

"Oftentimes seeming tragedies like my injury are clouds with a silver lining. After I'd rehabilitated my wrist I took careful stock of my physique, and regardless of how hard I tried to convince myself I was ready for the Junior Nationals, I just wasn't. I wasn't even close to being ready for it. I felt I needed a good, solid 15-18 pounds of additional muscle mass, better balanced physical proportions and more overall muscle hardness to be ready to win an open national-level title.

"So I dug in and did my homework for a solid eighteen months, always with that long-term goal of winning the Junior Nationals burning like a beacon in the distance. I *lived* bodybuilding 2½–3 hours per day, six days per week in the gym. I trained like a Trojan every workout—always going to *at least* 100 percent of my abilities—and I was making some incredible gains!

"I *ate* bodybuilding, too, carefully monitoring every gram of protein and every calorie I put into my mouth. And most importantly, I *thought* bodybuilding virtually every free hour of the day, seeing the beacon in the distance and constantly visualizing myself achieving my goal.

▼ **Vince Comerford** ➤

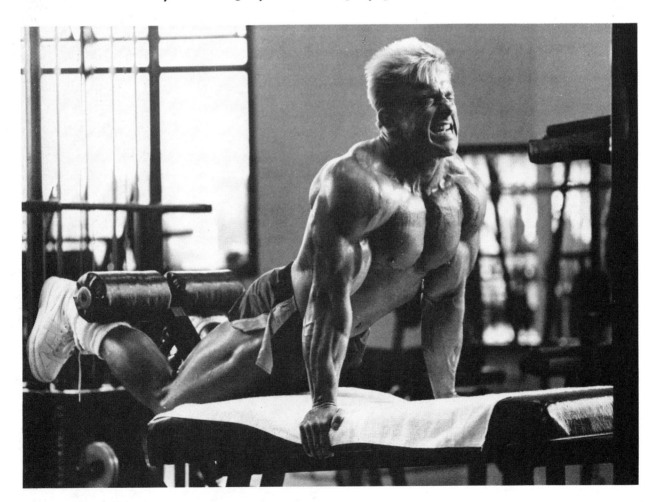

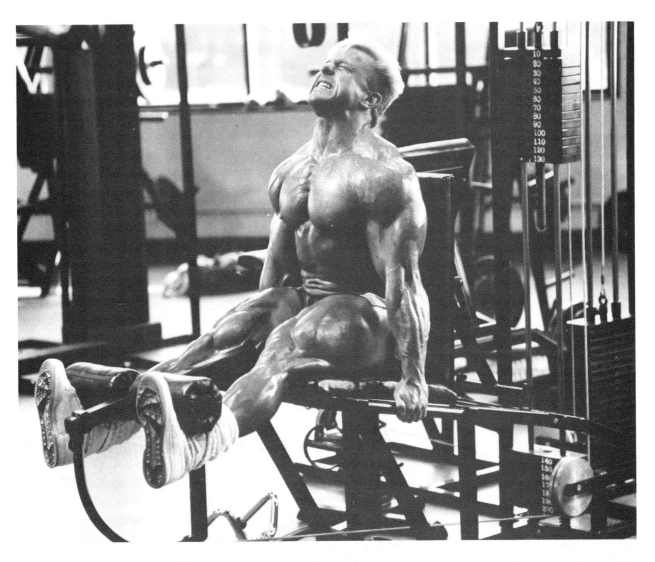

"By the time of the '82 Junior Nationals, I was *ready,* as totally ready as I could have possibly been. Believe me, I was R-E-A-D-Y.

"History shows I won the '82 Juniors, then came back a few weeks later to dominate the Heavyweight Class and also win the overall NPC National Championship at Madison Square Garden in New York City. A couple of weeks later in Bruges, Belgium, I added the IFBB Heavyweight World Championship to my list of victories for 1982. It would be tough to conceive of having a single better competitive year, but as I walked offstage at Bruges, I was already planning for 1983.

"My '83 long-range goals were to win the Night of the Champions, a prestigious pro show, then place in the top three at the Olympia later that year in Munich, West Germany. I prepared even more intensely than the previous year and achieved both goals, coming third behind Samir Bannout and Mohamed Makkawy at the Olympia, but ahead of three-time Mr. Olympia Frank Zane. To add a little icing to the cake, I also defeated John Terilli, Makkawy and many other top pros at the Caesars Palace Pro Invitational in Las Vegas, Nevada.

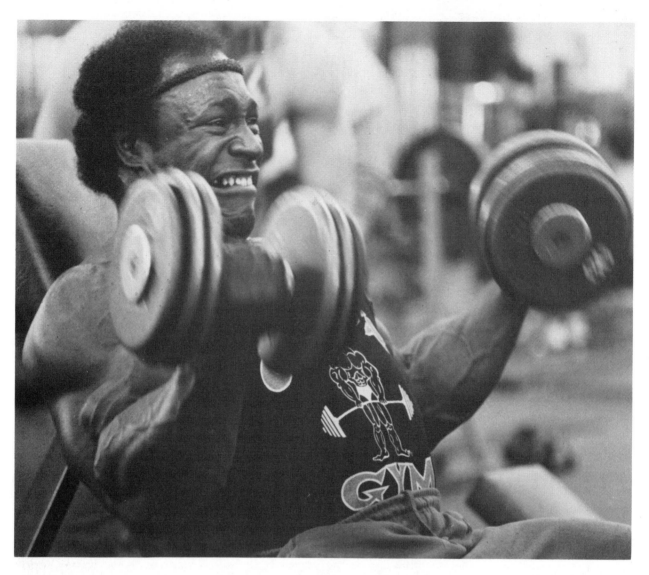

"My long-term goal for 1984 could be nothing other than to win my first Mr. Olympia title. I trained like a man possessed, particularly on arms and calves, monitoring every morsel of food I ate for the entire year. I was perfectly prepared mentally as well. History records 1984 as the year Lee Haney won his first Mr. Olympia title at a massive body weight of 242 pounds.

"Each year after that, my long-range goal was to win the Olympia again, particularly by improving my weaker areas every year.

"In order to win my fourth Olympia, the 1987 version in Göteborg, Sweden, I felt I still needed more leg mass, continued improvement in every other body part as well, and—if possible—an even more streamlined midsection. As in '86, I won the title, again with nine first place votes in every round. In fact, I was essentially compared only one time in the first round of judging, and it was all over. Now I'm looking forward to the '88 Olympia, with a weak point which needs improvement. You can bet it'll be up.

▲ The great Mr. Olympia Lee Haney at Gold's Gym, Toronto.

Lee Haney blasts ➤ his delts with dumbbell side laterals.

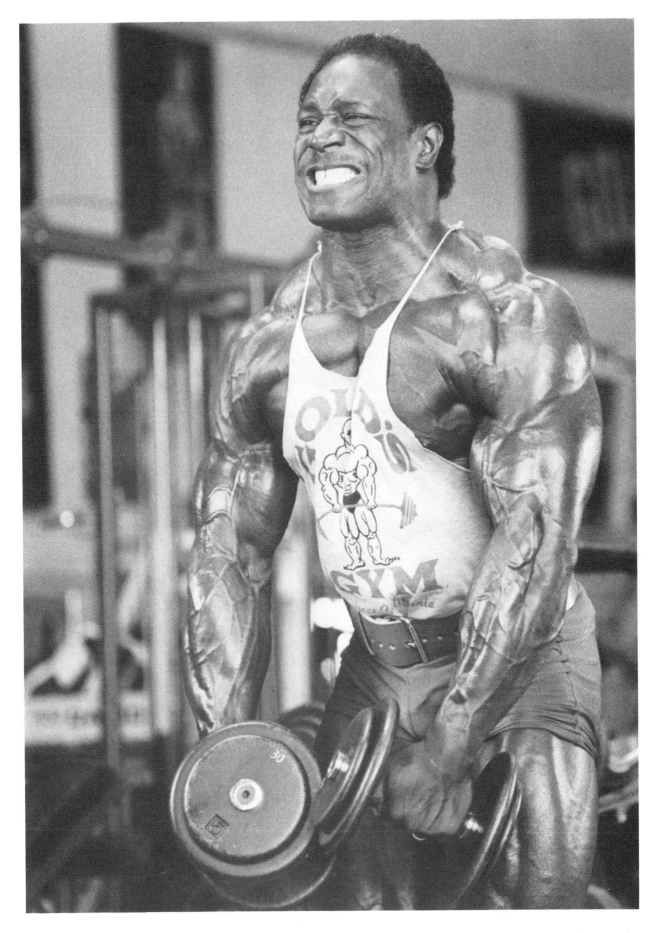

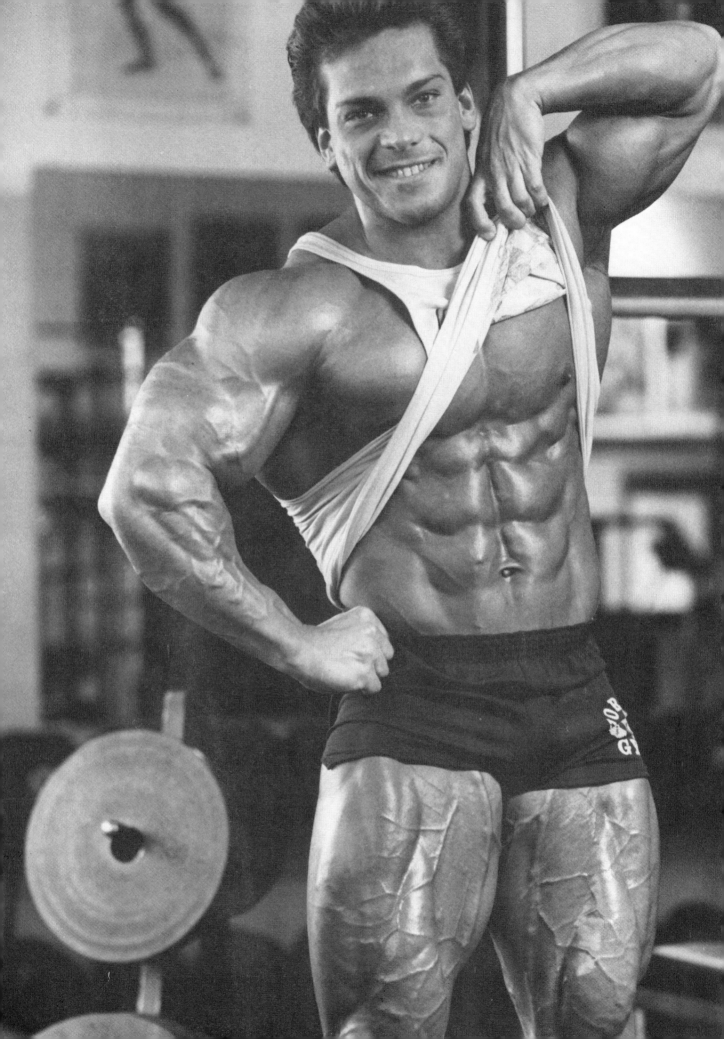

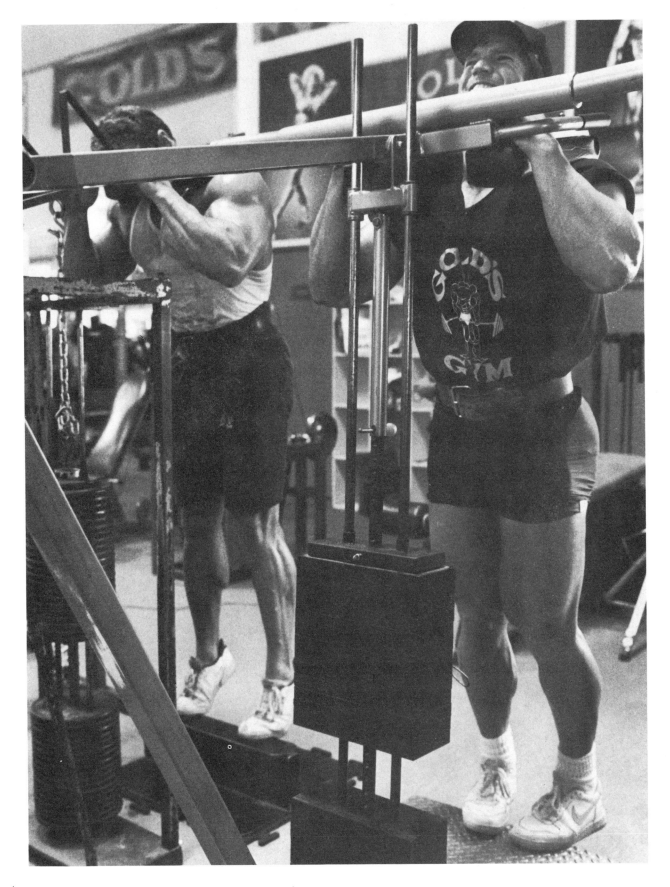

▲ Calf training at Gold's: D'Marko Blewett and Gary Strydom.

◄ Rich "Wonder Boy" Gaspari.

"The key thing in terms of goal setting for me over the years was to take things one logical, attainable step at a time. I would set my sights on a competition a year away, then virtually move heaven and earth to reach that goal. And when I won that show, I'd set my yearly, long-range goal at an even higher level of competition. In this way I stayed constantly motivated to continue improving enough each year to climb up the ladder to the Mr. Olympia title. It worked well for me, and it'll work well for you, too. Give my method of setting long-term goals a trial!"

While Lee Haney and scores of other top bodybuilders have been very successful in setting and attaining long-range goals in terms of competitions to be won, scores of other top men have set goals in terms of adding new inches of muscle mass to a weak body part and/or using a significant additional amount of weight in basic exercises that influence the weaker, lagging area(s). One of the best examples of this type of long-range goal setting has been provided by Vincent Comerford, who smashed his way to

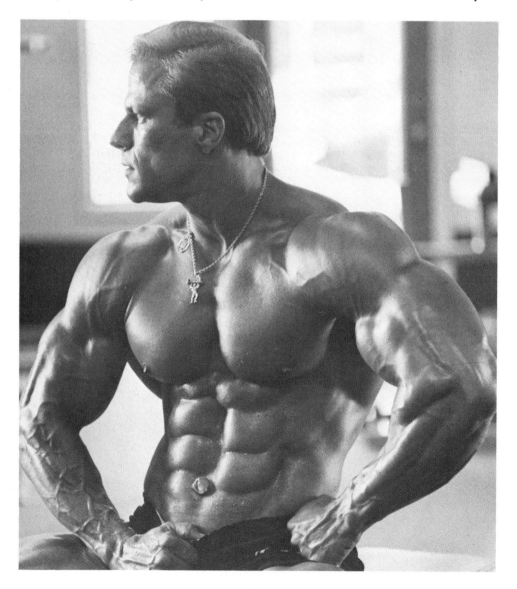

◄ These magnificent abs are the hallmark of John Hnatyschak's great physique.

Heavy dumbbell shrugs build powerful traps. ➤

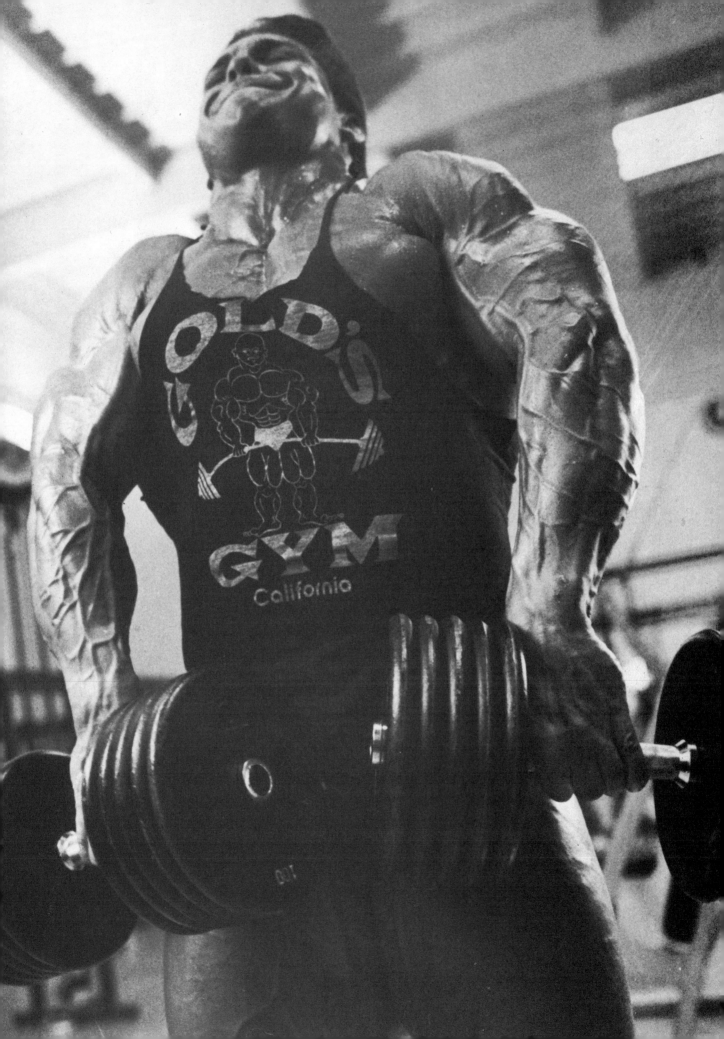

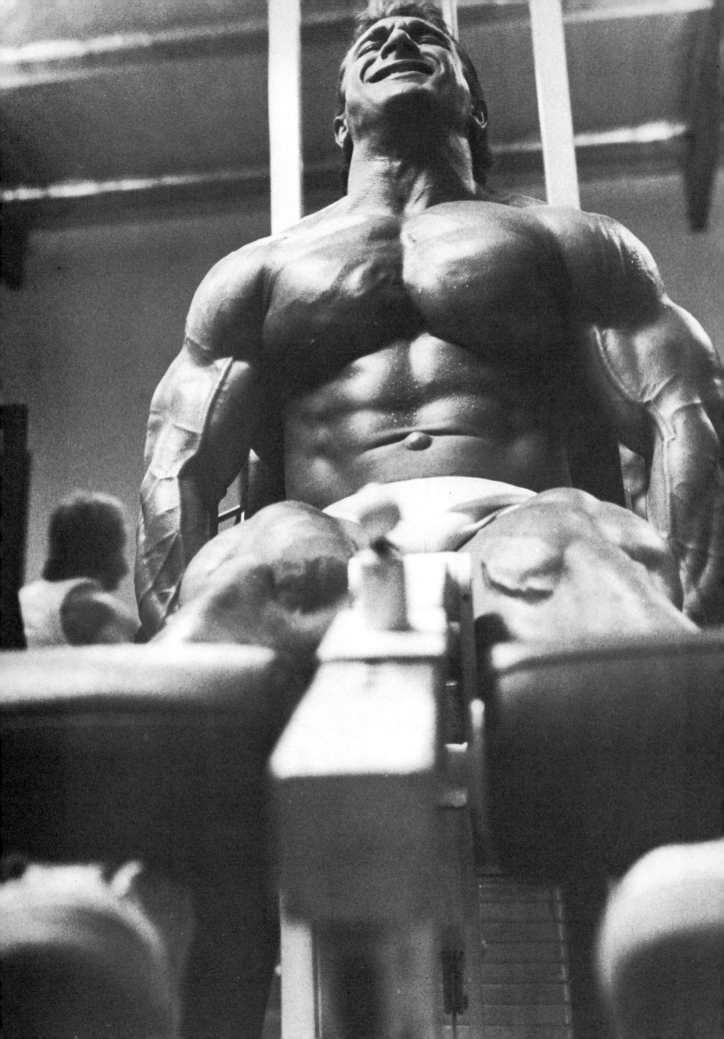

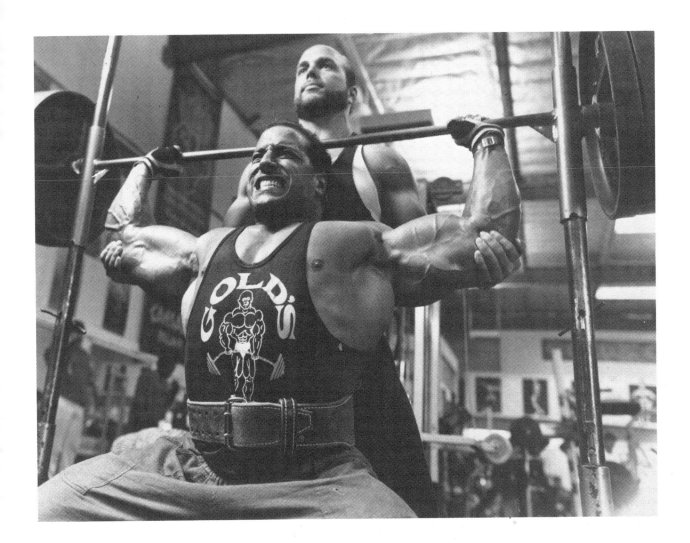

Mike Quinn is one of the most powerful men in bodybuilding.

Shane DiMora does thigh extensions.

a weight class win at the '87 NPC Nationals, when even the most avid afficionados of the sport would never have conceded the Middleweight National Championship to Comerford.

Vincent had an essentially world-class upper body for three to four years prior to winning Nationals. His arms were stupendously developed and the envy of many high-level IFBB pro bodybuilders. But Comerford's legs were pitifully weak, and this lack of development always kept Vincent out of the top positions at NPC national shows.

What did Vincent Comerford do to bring his woefully weak legs up to the level of the rest of his physique? He placed priority on training thighs and calves harder than any other body parts, and he used a different type of long-range goal setting quite effectively.

If you don't already understand the concept of muscle priority training, I should explain it to you. In general, when you are prioritizing a lagging muscle group, it must be bombed first in your workout when you have available maximum supplies of both physical energy and mental drive to expend on training the weak area with absolute maximum intensity. When your energy reserves have been depleted toward the end of a heavy training session, it would be physically impossible to train a lagging muscle group with the high degree of intensity possible at the beginning of a workout.

The converse side of muscle priority training is also true—you must train naturally responsive muscle groups with lesser intensity and toward the end of a workout. In rare cases, when a body part is overwhelmingly well developed, you should actually suspend training it for several months, banking the energy you would normally have used to work it for expenditure on weaker sections of your physique. Only six to eight weeks of hard training on highly responsive muscle complexes will bring them back up to their original level.

A third refinement of muscle priority training—and the one Vincent Comerford used to great advantage on his quads and hamstrings—is to set aside training days each week to bomb the bejesus out of a single very weak area. Vincent's legs were weakest, so he trained them by themselves once every four days, doing quads alone in the morning and hamstrings by themselves in the evening part of his double-split routine. Two other

▼ Upright rowing with 225 pounds is child's play for the powerful Mike Quinn. ➤

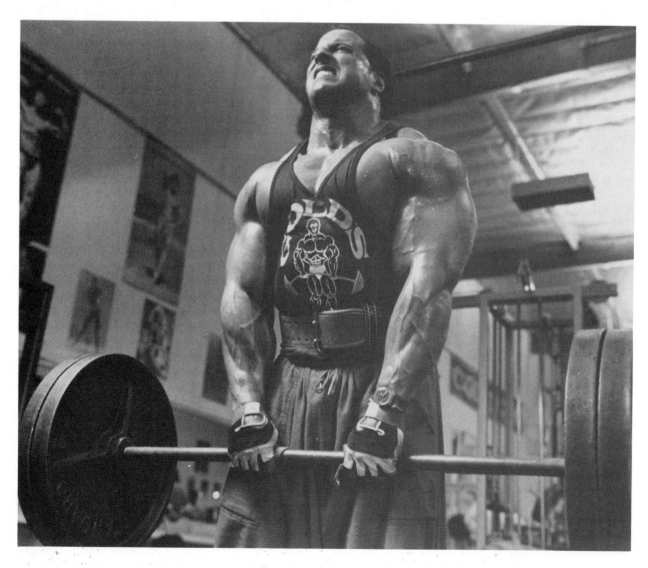

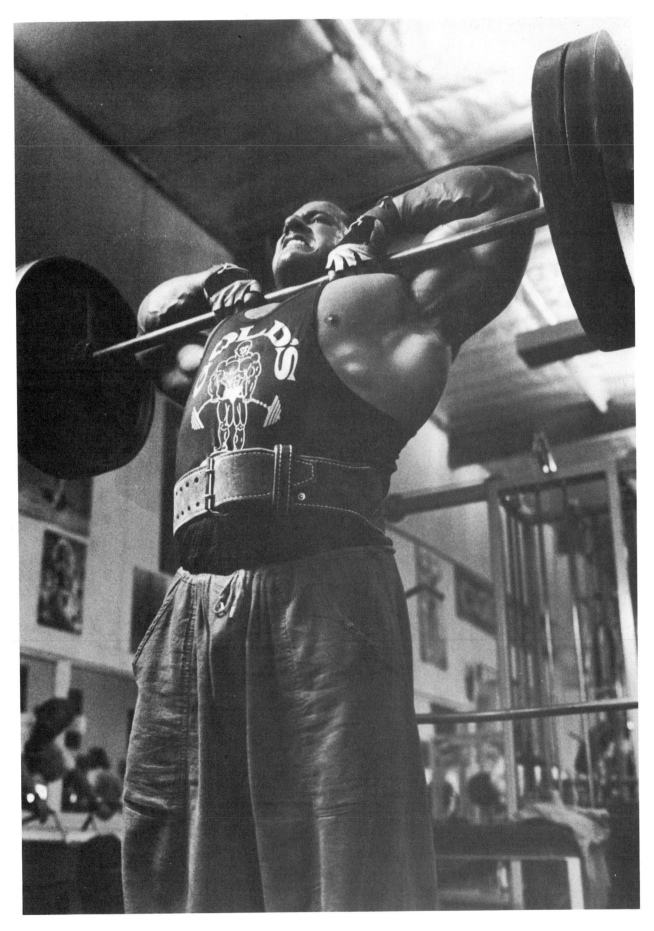

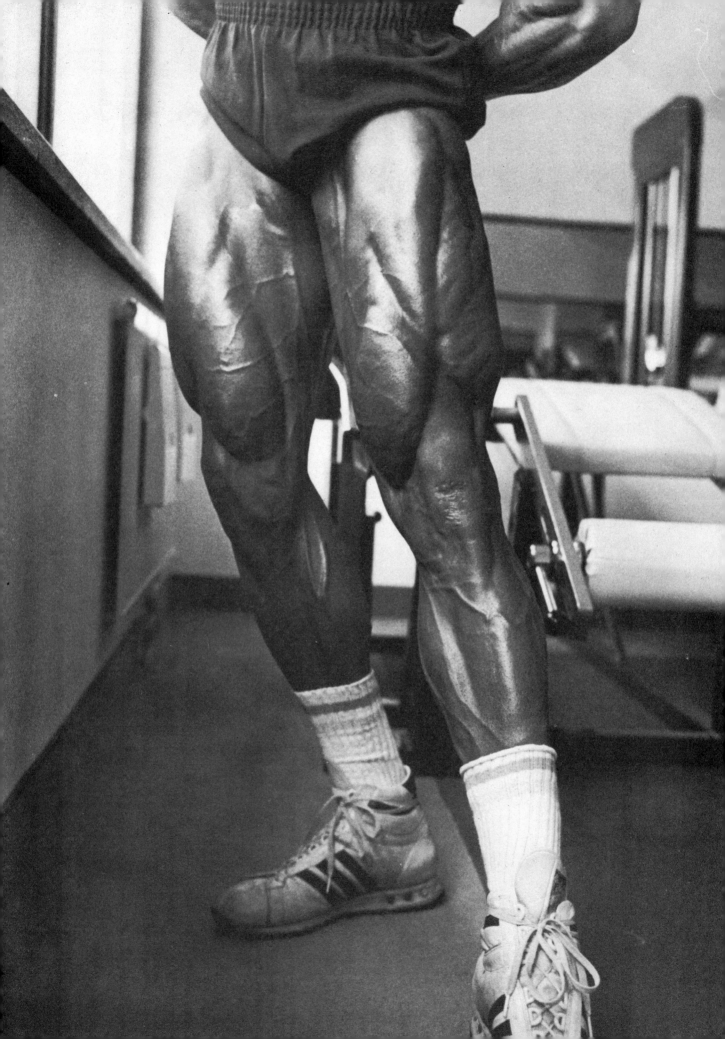

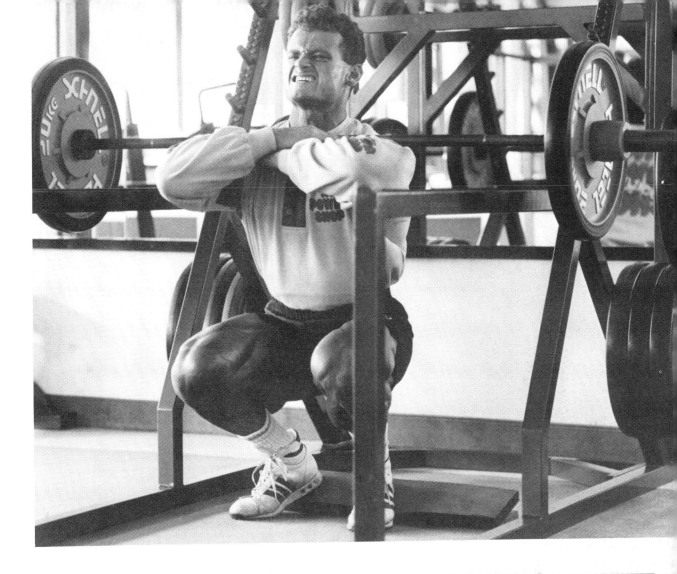

Front squats are the most demanding frontal thigh exercise.

The hamstrings. ➤

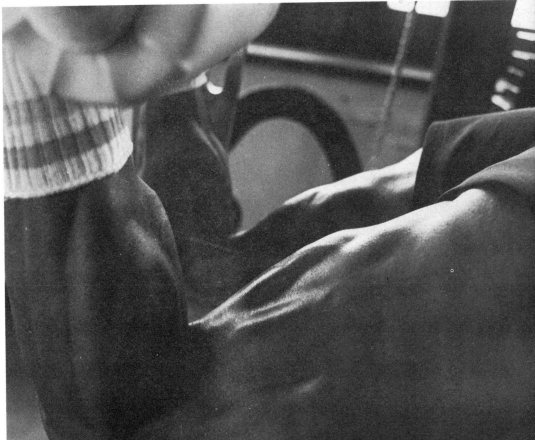

◄ Ripped frontal thigh muscles.

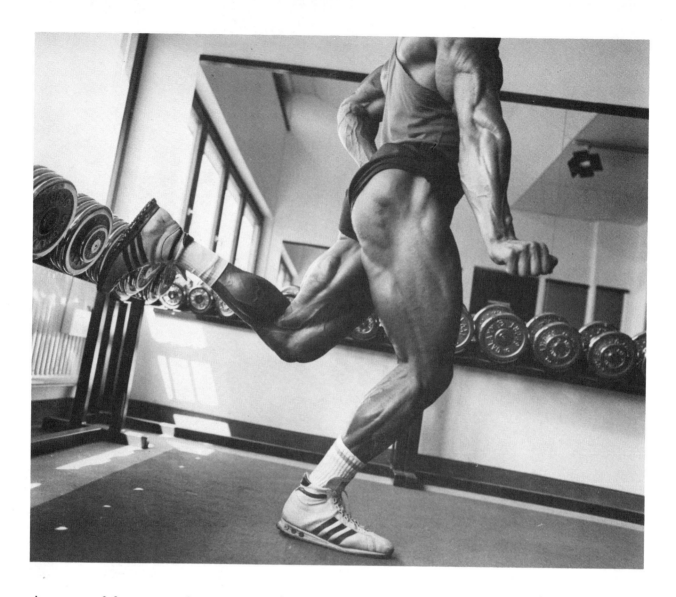

The hamstrings.

days out of four were devoted to the remaining body parts, with calves only trained alone in the evening twice each four days, more or less every other day. The fourth day was a full rest day, and the cycle began repeating on the fifth day.

Where did long-term goal setting come into the picture? Vincent knew full squats were the key to adding mass and contour to his quads, so he set as one yearly, long-term goal increasing his squat (going down far enough for his hamstrings to rest firmly against his calves at the bottom of each repetition) poundage for ten reps on his top set by 100 pounds. And through use of short-term goal setting (discussed in the next section) he was able to increase his squat poundage for reps by the full 100 pounds. In the process he added 2 inches to the girth of his thighs.

Comerford followed a similar method in his leg curl and stiff-legged dead-lift poundages, exercises which would greatly enhance the development of his hamstrings and glutes. To make a long story short, within two years of setting long-term goals in terms of poundage for his quads and hamstrings exer-

The fabulous abs of Bertil Fox. ➤

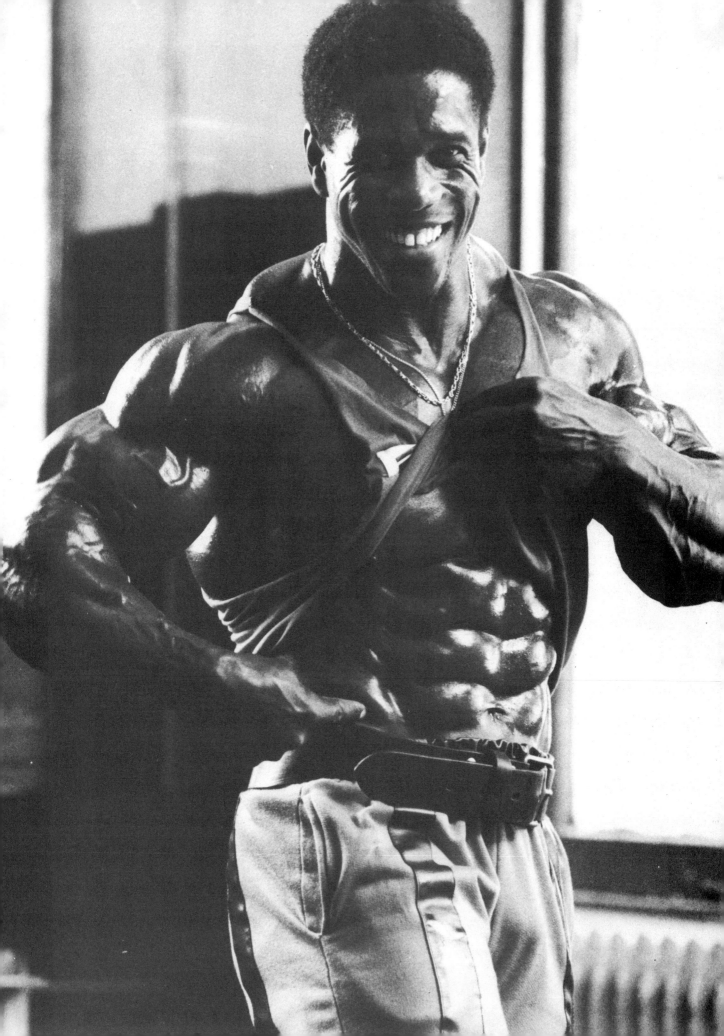

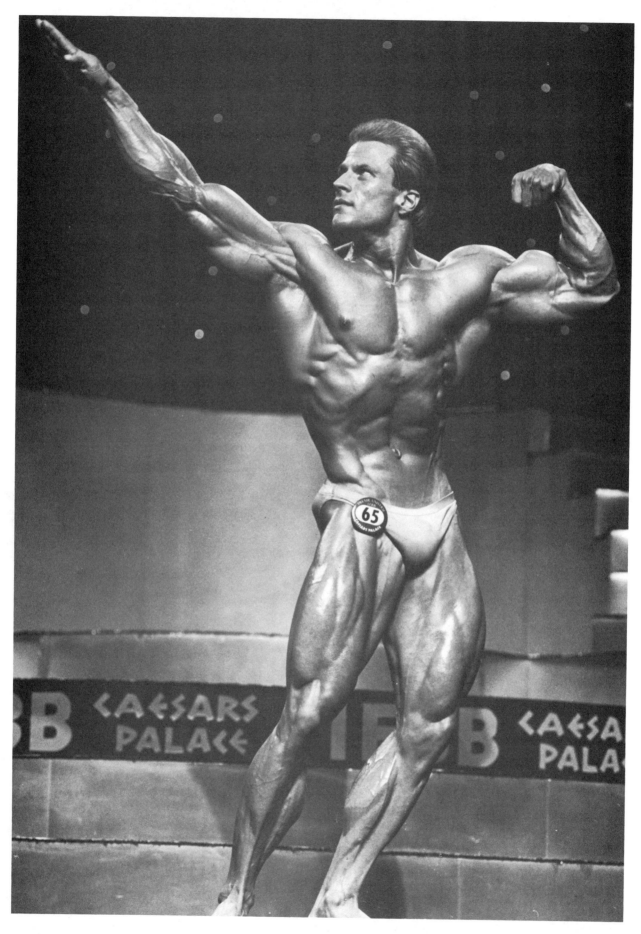

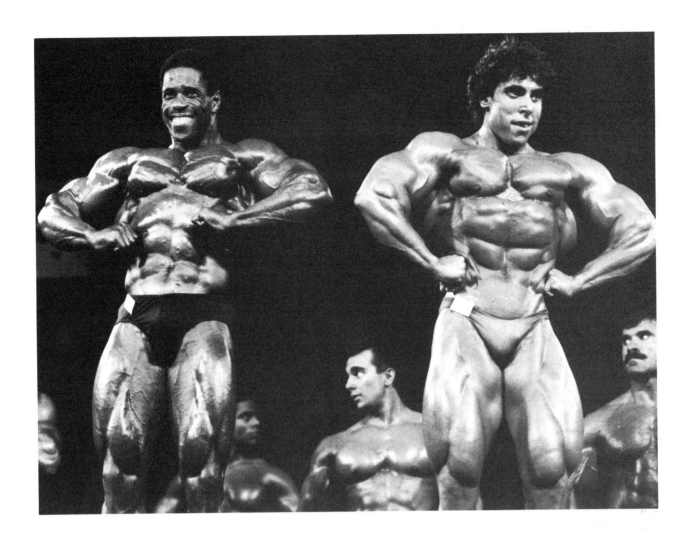

cises—plus consistently bombing away on his improving calves—Vincent Comerford had brought his leg development into perfect balance with the rest of his physique. He easily won the 1987 NPC National Middleweight Championship and has become a highly successful IFBB pro bodybuilder.

### Short-range Goals

Yearly long-term goals should be subdivided into short-range goals. Normally it's best to set short-term goals at monthly intervals (twelve per year), although some very successful competitive bodybuilders set short-range goals at weekly intervals (meaning there are fifty-two of these short-term goals per year).

I interviewed leading pro bodybuilder Mike Christian (he's won the NPC Heavyweight and Overall National Championships, was victorious at the IFBB World Championships and placed in the top three at the Mr. Olympia show) about short-range goal setting: "Overall, I'm a big believer in setting, achieving and resetting goals at even higher levels. Goal setting is one of the main reasons why I have risen so high in the bodybuilding ranks over the years.

"Like every other top bodybuilder, my ultimate goal is to become Mr. Olympia, and I can absolutely guarantee I'll win that title one day, come Haney, hell or high water. All of my long-term goals are set in terms of improving a weak body part or two in the off-season. And each time I bring up one lagging muscle group, my physique improves drastically. The hallmark of all great pro bodybuilders is perfect proportional balance between all of the various body parts. We all have mass, deep cuts and varying degrees of body symmetry, so it's relative proportional balance which wins it or loses it for each of us at an Olympia.

"Deltoids are a very well-developed body part for me, but to illustrate how I'd use short-range goal setting to improve a weak area, let's say my delts *are* weak and that I'm determined to bring them up to the level of the rest of my physique within one year's time.

"I believe—indeed, most top bodybuilders believe—there is a direct correlation between training weights and the mass of the muscles which move a particular weight in good form for reps. Simply put, being able to do presses behind neck and standing barbell upright rows with heavier and heavier weights will make my deltoids progressively more massive. So my entire goal for the year will be to increase poundages on those two basic exercises which build up my deltoid mass.

"For the sake of illustration, let's say that at the beginning of the year, I can do six reps of seated presses behind the neck with 225 pounds and six reps of upright rows with 185 pounds in good form. So I set as my long-range, yearly goal adding 40 pounds to my presses and 30 pounds to my rows. If a bodybuilder trains hard and consistently—and is very motivated—these are reasonable goals to shoot for.

"The problem really lies in your brain's unwillingness to accept such large figures for increased poundage on each movement. So I fake it out by breaking these yearly goals down into smaller—and more believable—short-term monthly goals. Adding 5 pounds per month (it even *sounds* easy) to presses would give me a 60-pound gain in one year, 20 pounds more than I'm shooting for. And to reach a 30-pound increase in rows over a one-year period I'd only need to increase my training poundage by a measly 2½ pounds per month! Any pencil-neck geek could do that, right?

"All long-range goals can be subdivided into many smaller short-range goals which are easier to comprehend mentally and accomplish physically. But step by step, they all add up. Step by step, they take you through the low amateur ranks, through the national amateur shows, and finally into the pro shows. And it's *easy*."

Every top bodybuilder uses these goal-setting techniques to more completely focus his or her mind on the task at hand, which is systematically improving a physique until it reaches its maximum potential. Simply let Lao-tzu show you the easy way to the top!

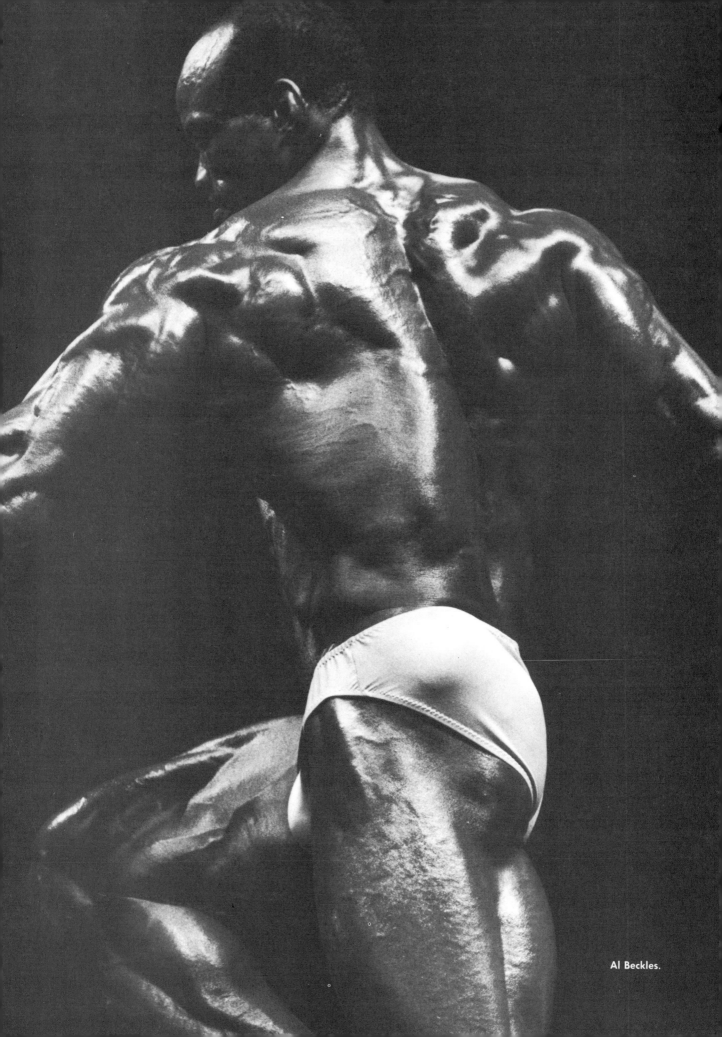

Al Beckles.

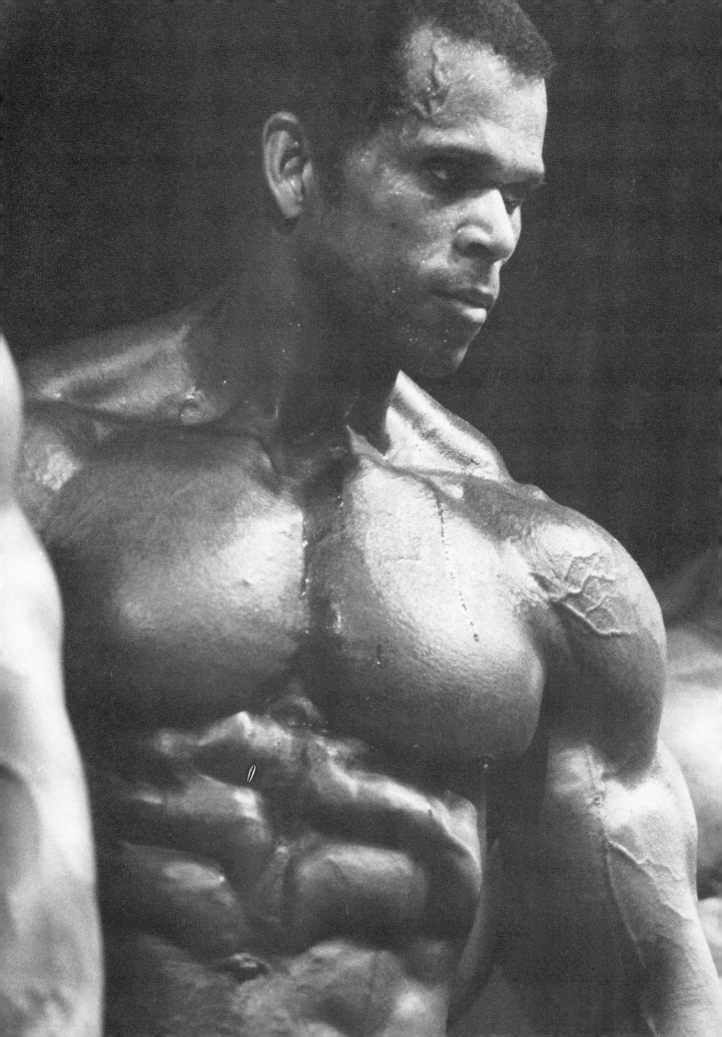

# 3

# Concentration

**A**very top bodybuilder has pinpoint mental concentration on his working muscles during every repetition of each set of his workout. He is able to concentrate so intently on the contractions and extensions of the working muscles during a set that everything happening in the gym is blocked out. Someone could ask him a question in mid set, but he wouldn't hear a word.

Shawn Ray (California and National Champion) talks about concentration ability: "All of the champions have it, just as a natural consequence of several years of hard, consistent training. But why should an enthusiastic young bodybuilder wait years for concentration skills to develop on their own? Why not work at developing good concentration early in your body-building involvement?

"The first step to learning proper workout concentration is to study an anatomy chart so you know where you should feel each repetition of all the exercises in your routine. Then when you do each set, try to visualize that muscle—or those muscles—powerfully contracting and then extending under a heavy load on every rep. This is most easily done at first in front

◄ Serge Nubret, one of the all-time masters of Zen bodybuilding.

of a mirror. But even without a mirror, try to feel every rep in the muscles you are working with each exercise.

"When you first start working on your powers of concentration, you'll find your mind quickly skipping off on to some other topic. You'll be able to think about anything but your workouts. But every time your mind skips off the working muscles, you should attempt to immediately force it back on those muscles. Each succeeding workout you'll find your mind skipping off less quickly and less often, until finally you have developed great workout concentration.

"How long should this process take? It took me about eighteen months to perfect my own concentration ability, which I feel is about average for a young bodybuilder. With consistent practice on your concentration, you should have it up to a high enough level in one or two years. And then you'll be getting great results from all of your workouts!"

1987 IFBB Amateur World Champion Luiz Freitas. ➤

▼ Phil Hill.

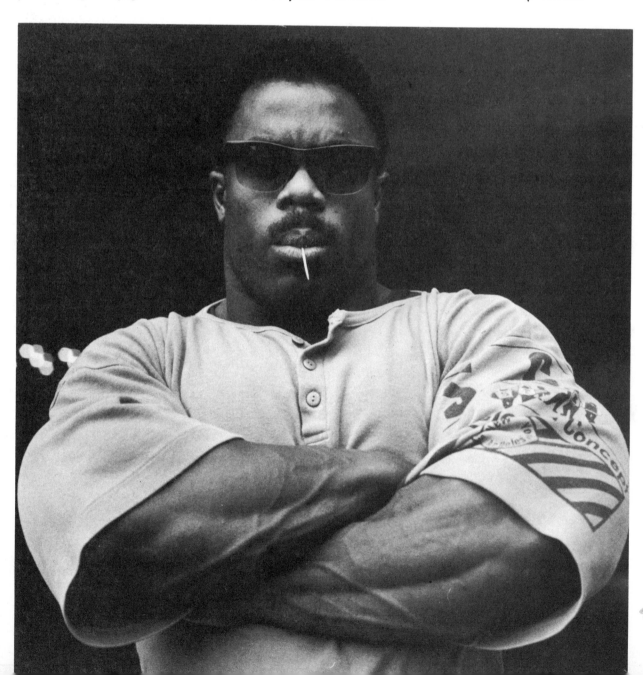

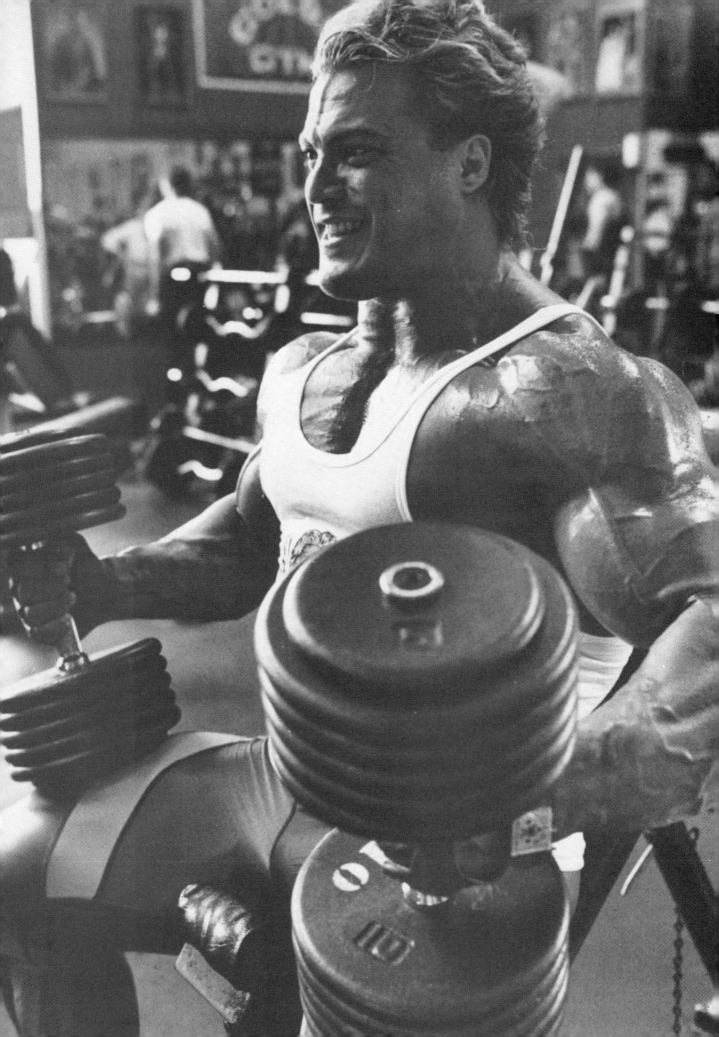

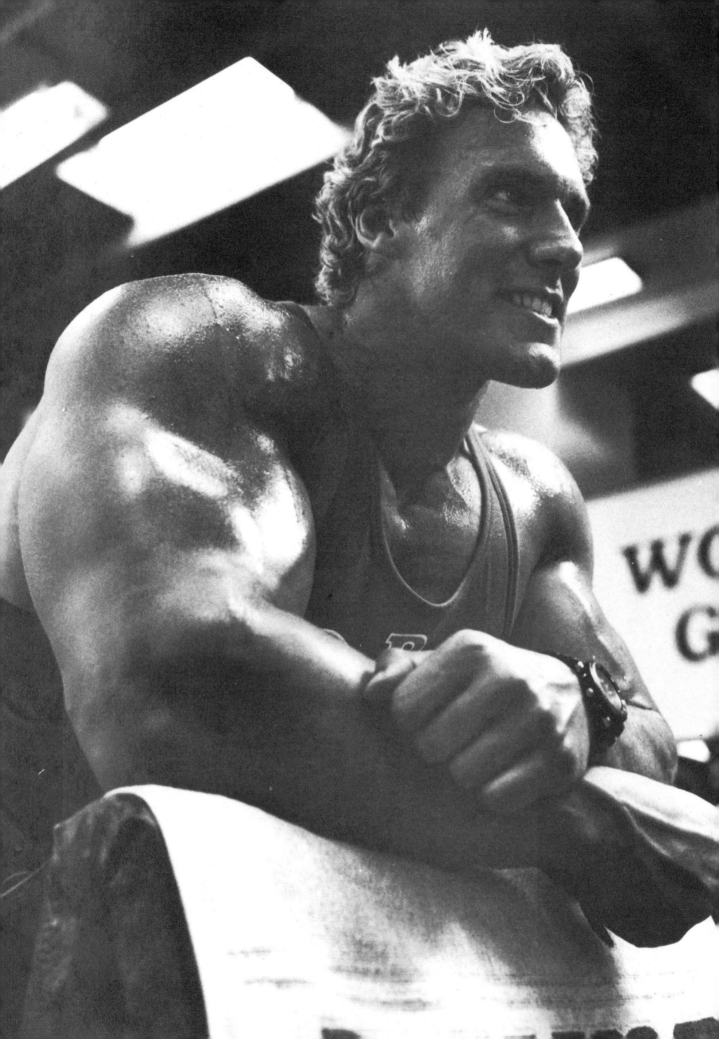

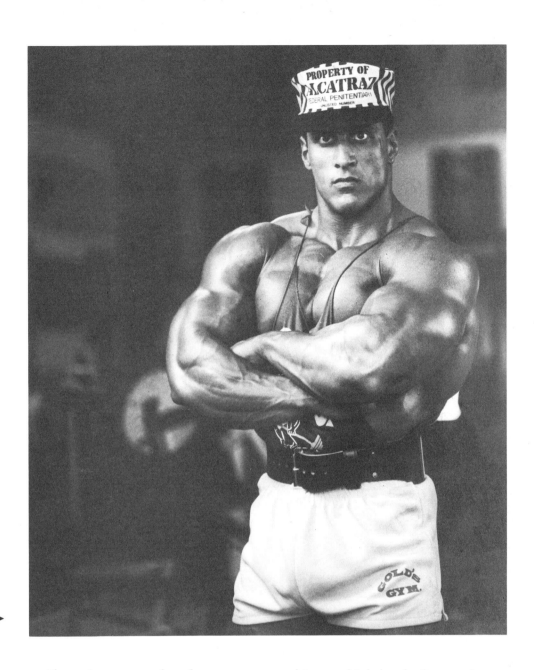

The amazing Mike ▶
Quinn.

◀ Ralf Moeller's work-
outs begin in his
mind.

There is a somewhat faster way to achieve a high level of mental concentration—meditation. Frank Zane always gets up early enough each day
to meditate for 20–30 minutes prior to his 6:00 A.M. workout. In this way
Zane marshals his mental energies and focuses them exclusively on his
workout. Zane's level of mental concentration is as deep as anyone's in
the sport.

Meditation to develop better workout concentration is *not* some type of
New Age hokum. It can be a vital part of Zen Buddhism, but in our sense
it will be used merely as a means of centering the mind on a specific task,
concentration on the working muscles during a set. It definitely works well
to develop better concentration as long as you believe in it and work at
the process. It has worked quite well for Zane and many other top bodybuilders.

The most basic goal of meditation is to calm your mind and relax your body. This is called stabilization meditation. At successively higher levels of meditation you will be able to improve mental concentration and even gain enlightenment about the hazy inner workings of your own mind.

Under normal circumstances your mind is abuzz with random thoughts. These thoughts are almost like electrical sparks flying off an overcharged electrical pole. Another way to conceptualize this is to think of your mind as the crenellated surface of an ocean, the peak of each wave being a separate thought. The surface of the ocean is alive with wave crests just as your mind experiences a myriad of thoughts, each tumbling over the others. With proper meditation, you can calm the surface of the most storm-driven ocean.

Meditation practice should take place as regularly as possible, preferably every day. You should meditate in a quiet place, where you won't be interrupted while meditating. Emphasis should be on comfort, so try to have a pillow or cushion to sit on when meditating.

In classic meditation, you should be sitting in a full lotus position. In this position, your legs should be crossed and your feet placed soles upward on the opposite legs. Your spine should be held straight, one vertebra stacked on the one beneath it, just like you would stack a column of quarters. Rest your hands loosely in your lap, and you have achieved the perfect meditation position.

Very few bodybuilders are flexible enough to achieve a full lotus position, so you will probably have to make some adaptations to this posture. It's probably best to merely cross your lower legs with the edges of your feet resting on the floor, the soles of your feet facing outward away from each other. It's essential, however, that your spine be held straight, since this is the only position in which you can sit comfortably for 20–30 minutes. You can still rest your hands in your lap, but do so in the most comfortable possible position.

When you first start meditating, you will find it easier to accomplish with your eyes closed. As you grow more advanced, you might want to experiment with holding your eyes slightly open and downcast, since allowing in some light will keep you from drifting off into sleep. While it will be a good idea to fall asleep while practicing visualization, it's a negative happening when you are meditating.

Emphasis should be on comfort and relaxation when meditating, so feel free to make whatever modifications you need in the foregoing procedure. There is plenty of room for individual idiosyncracies, as long as you are comfortable.

The best place to start in meditation is in focusing your attention on your breathing. Sit erect and concentrate your mind on each inhalation and

Shawn Ray. ➤

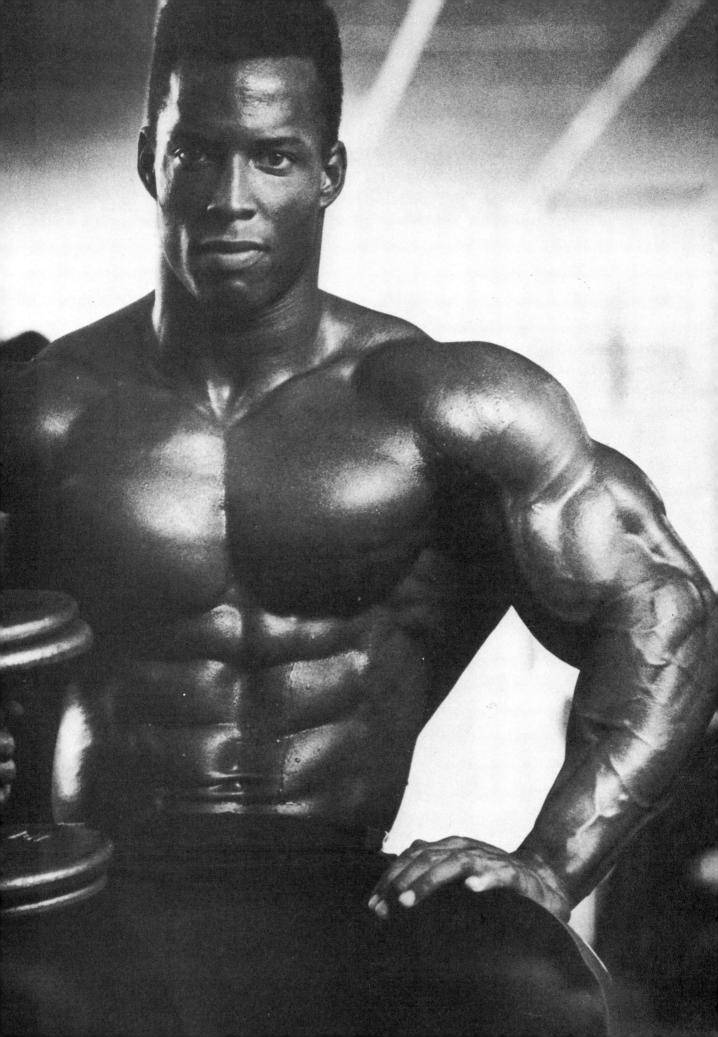

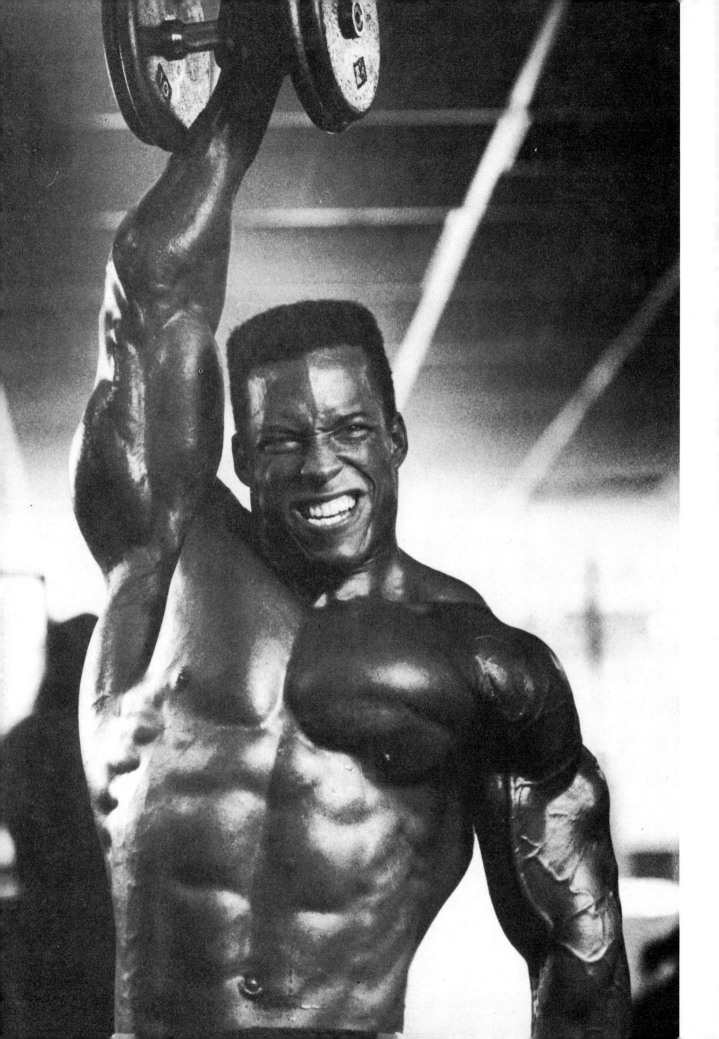

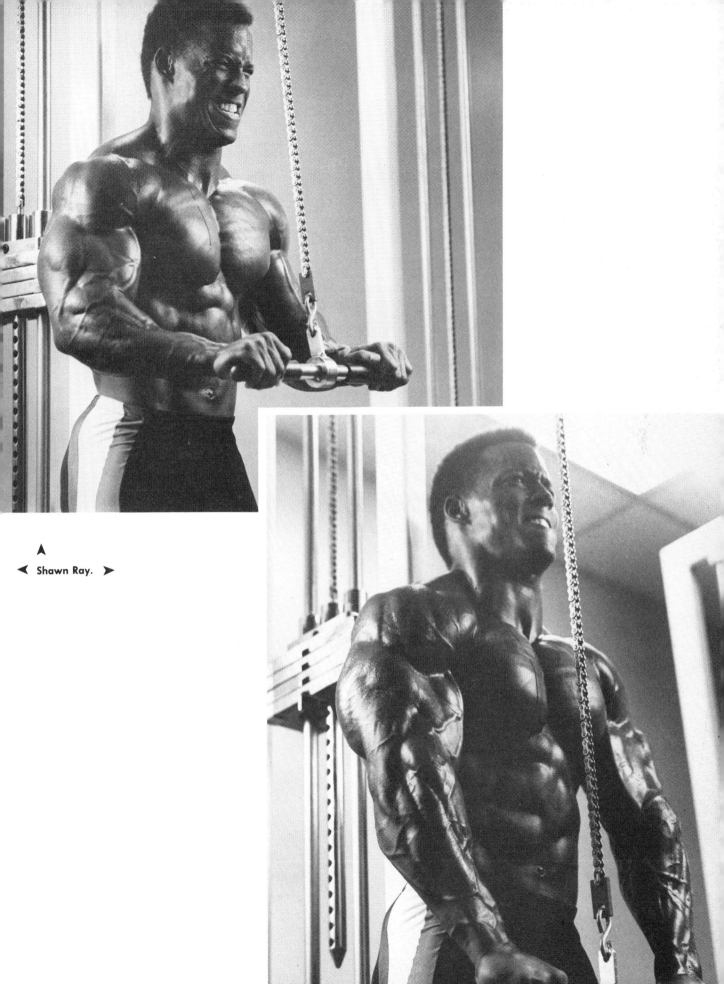

Shawn Ray.

exhalation, counting the inhalations and relaxing each time you exhale. Count slowly up to ten, one count on each inhalation. Whenever you reach ten, or lose count, start back at one.

At first you'll lose count a lot, an indication that your mental focus is not fully concentrated. But by disciplining yourself to start back at one each time you lose count, you'll find that you can soon count inhalations in sets of ten for up to 30 minutes. And with some work you'll be able to do sets of twenty to thirty inhalations without losing track of the count.

This is a very simple exercise, but it builds concentration ability relatively quickly. And your concentration will develop more quickly if you work consistently on this exercise.

There are many other meditation methods. One, which you may have heard about, is the use of a sonic stimulus, a mantra. The easiest one to use is the sound "ooommm," repeated over and over in sets of ten or more. You can also focus on a candle flame or some other visual point.

There are many excellent books on meditation which you might read to learn more about this fascinating subject. The one I've personally found easiest to understand is Kathleen McDonald's *How to Meditate—A Practical Guide.* It's not an easy book to find in bookshops, but well worth the search.

Shawn Ray. ➤

▼ Graeme Lancefield psychs himself before a heavy set of dumbbell bench presses.

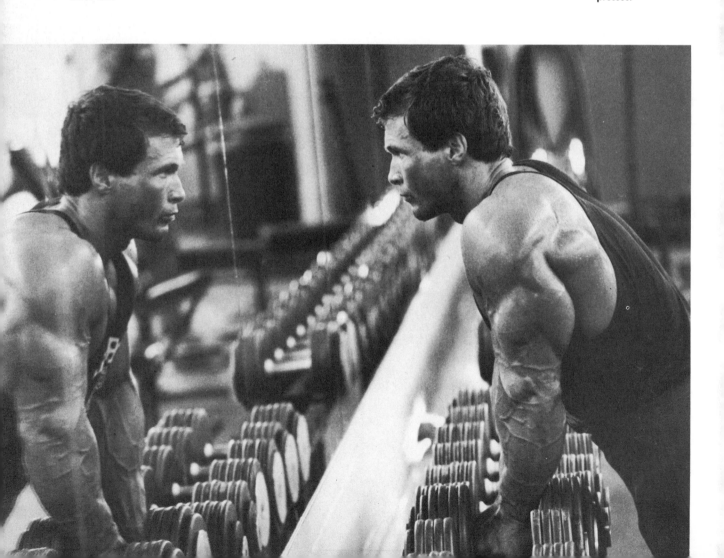

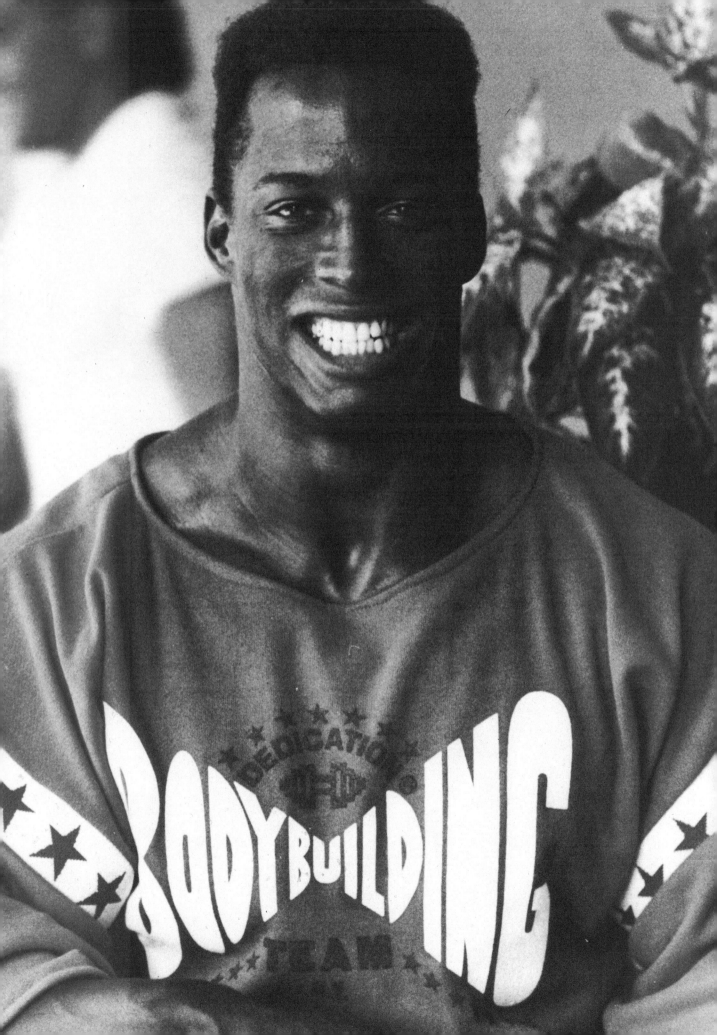

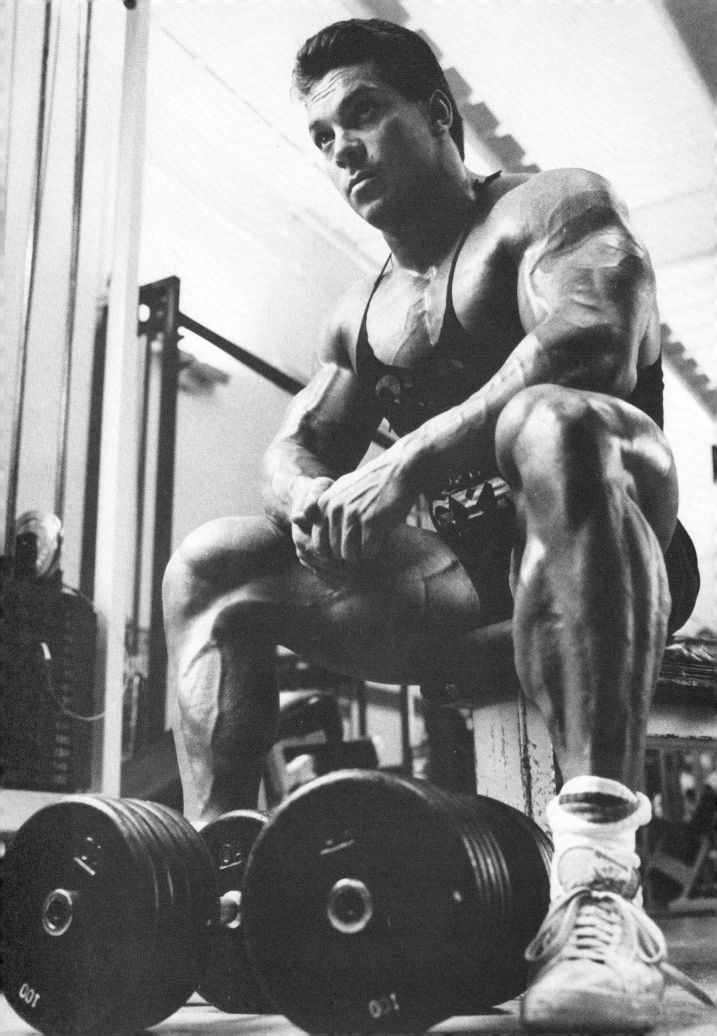

# 4

# Self-Actualization Through Visualization

**A**ny psychologist will tell you that your subconscious mind is far more powerful than your conscious mind. It is far more logical in the decisions it reaches, and it does not react to emotional issues. If you can harness the power of your subconscious mind to aid your bodybuilding efforts, you will be positively amazed at how much progress can be made in such a short period of time to improve your muscle mass, balance your proportions and develop a high degree of muscle density and muscularity. Properly harnessed, your subconscious mind can even greatly improve your posing and stage presence once you are in competition.

Psychologists talk about a process called "self-actualization," in which a young man or woman yearns to become a great mathematician, musician, athlete, or whatever, yearns to such a degree that he or she fantasizes constantly about living such a life. This fantasizing actually convinces the subconscious mind—after a long period of time, but nonetheless much as you might program a computer—to believe the person already has achieved the fantasized status.

In pure self-actualization, the programmed subconscious mind makes an

◀ Gaspari! The ultimate Zen bodybuilder.

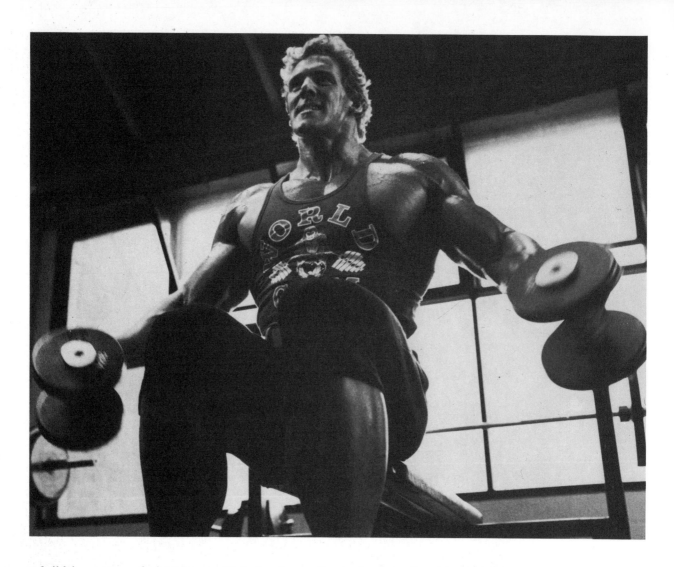

infallible series of decisions which leads easily and naturally toward the profession or skill for which it has been programmed. It becomes easy, for example, to sit down at a piano and practice a Mozart concerto over and over for 6–8 hours at a time. It makes the study of a human anatomy textbook a joyful experience, rather than the drudgery most premed students experience when reading the same book. And it becomes easy to maintain the tight low-fat/low-calorie diet every bodybuilder must maintain in order to reach contest condition.

You can't beat this kind of mental programming, because anyone can achieve it with a minimum of instruction, and it works well for virtually everyone. It's a crying shame that more bodybuilders fail to get in touch with neglected, powerful sections of their minds. Self-actualization works wonderfully well for everyone willing to work at it, so let's get started on developing and utilizing our subconscious minds to greatly improve our physiques.

Random daydreaming can lead to self-actualization, but it's a very weak method compared to consistent mental visualization. And all this involves is lying down in a comfortable position each night and creatively day-

◄ Seated side dumb-
bell laterals for
wide shoulders. ►

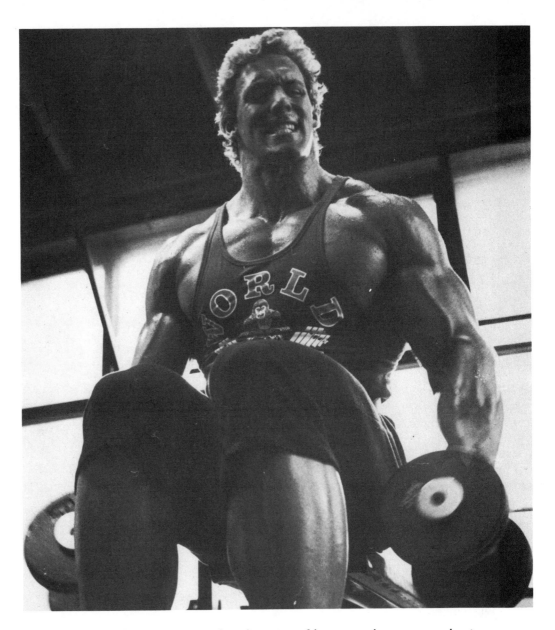

dreaming, conjuring up a visualized image of how you *know* your physique will look a few months from now. It's a very pleasant process, and you'll rapidly become addicted (in a very positive way, of course) to it. But the greater your addiction to visualization, the more it will help you to achieve the physique you've dreamed about having for years.

The following five requisites to effective visualization must be observed:

- Freedom from distractions (e.g., loud music in the next apartment, an interruption from your mate, etc.)
- A calm and relaxed position in bed
- A dark room
- Relative quiet
- At least 30 minutes in which to practice visualization (This amount of time will be greatly reduced as you become more adept at the technique.)

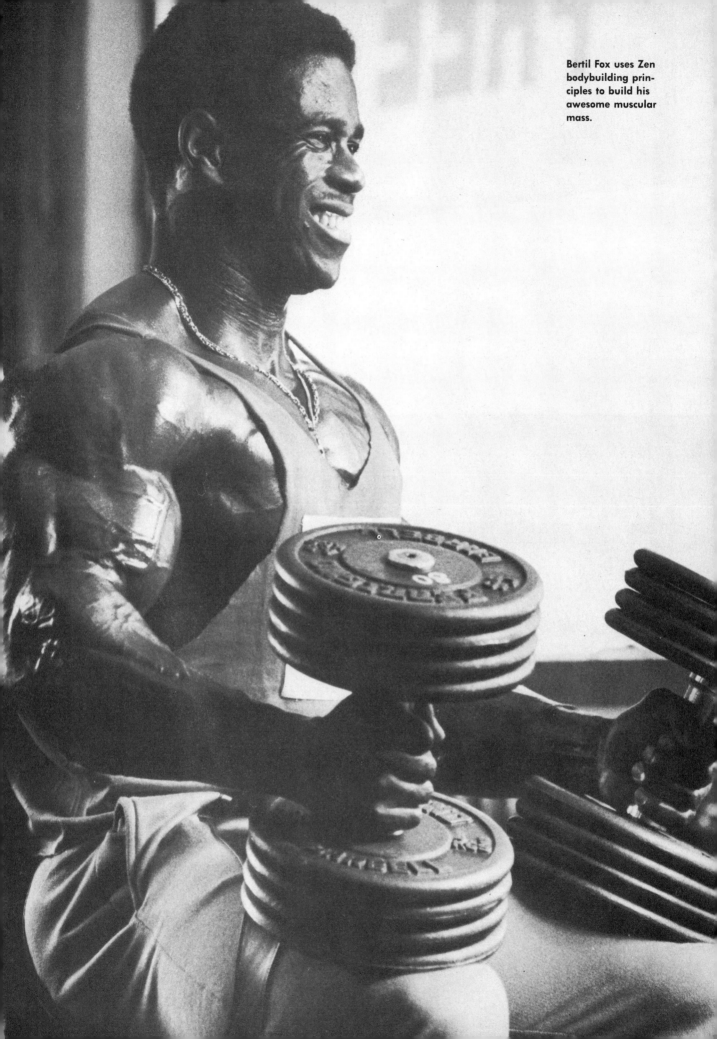

Bertil Fox uses Zen bodybuilding principles to build his awesome muscular mass.

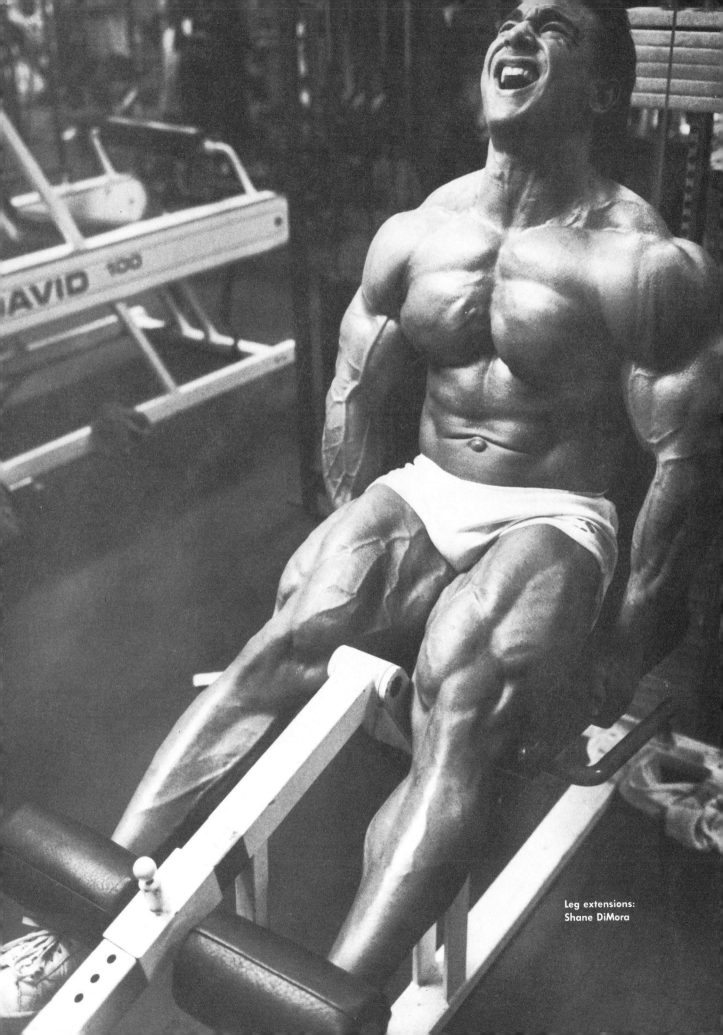

Leg extensions:
Shane DiMora

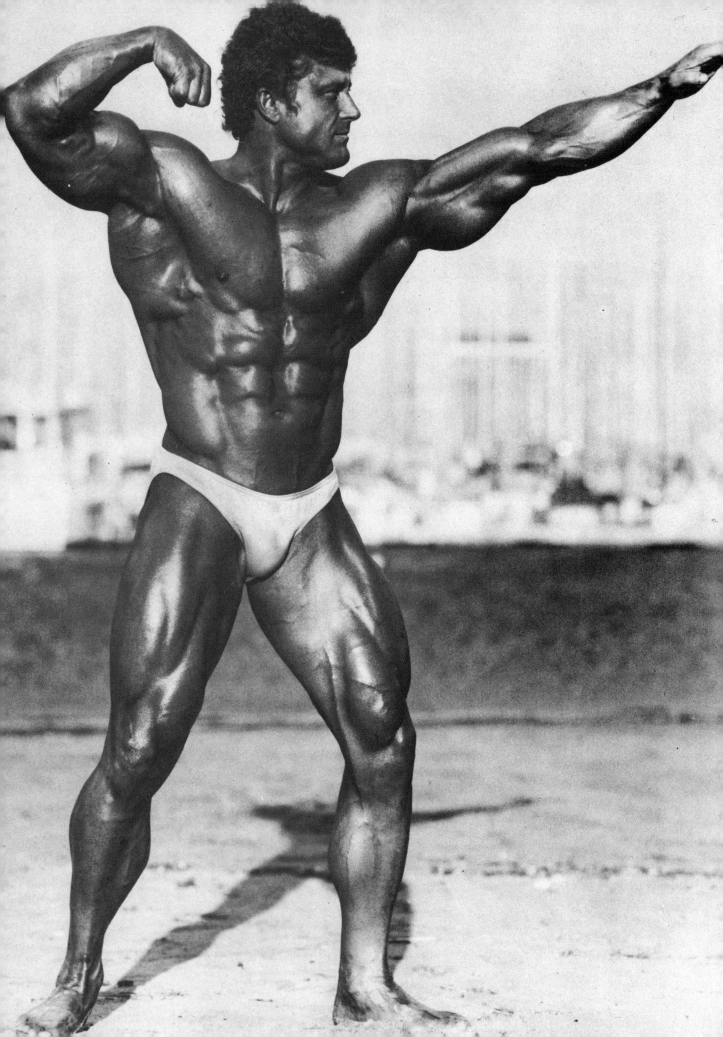

Given these five requirements, I feel it is best to practice mental visualization when you are in bed, relaxed and almost ready to fall asleep. Indeed, you may actually fall asleep while visualizing how you plan to soon look, but falling asleep during the process actually helps your subconscious mind become more deeply programmed with the mentally generated image you have conjured up.

Let's start our discussion of visualization by learning how to put your body and mind in the correct attitude. First turn out the bedroom lights and lie on your back in bed, your legs spread slightly apart and your arms lying on the bed at your sides. Place one pillow under your head and neck, a second one beneath your knees. Your body is now in a good position for it to become completely relaxed.

The best way to relax your body is through a process called "fractional relaxation," which amounts to concentrating on relaxing each body part by itself in a sequence which ultimately leads to a fully relaxed, full-body state. At first, fractional relaxation will require as many as 30–40 minutes

Luiz Freitas "spots" ➤
his training part-
ner Tom Dunn.

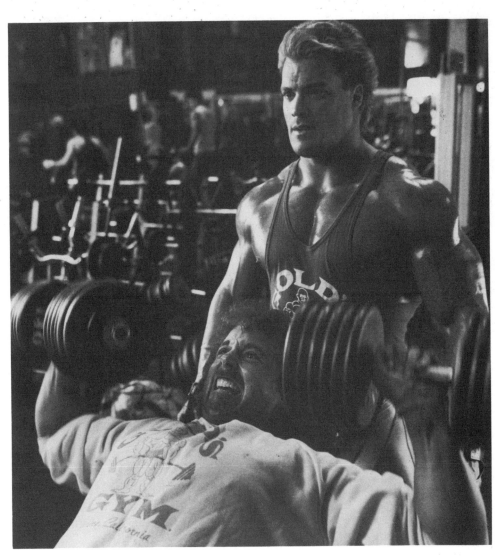

◄ The remarkable
Frank Richard
made the greatest
comeback in body-
building history.

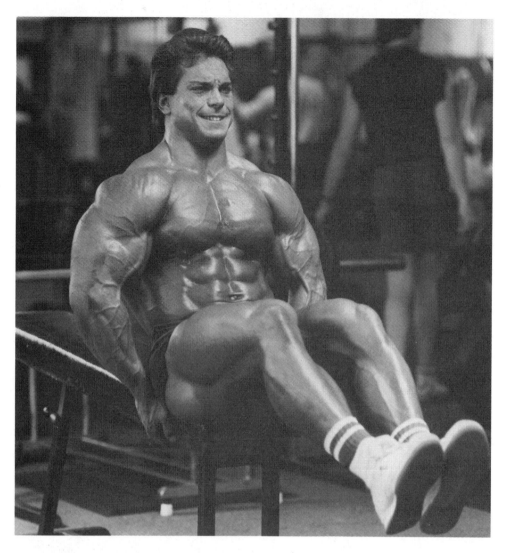

◄ Seated knee-ups with Gaspari.

to complete, but with practice you will soon be able to relax your entire body in less than 10 minutes.

Start by breathing slowly and rhythmically, concentrating on relaxing your left foot and ankle. Usually this is most easily done if you first tense all of the muscles of the area on which you're working for 10–15 seconds, then totally relax them. Repeat the procedure on your right foot and ankle. Continue up your body in sequence, doing your calves, hamstrings, quadriceps, buttocks, lower back, abdominals, middle back, pectorals, trapezius muscles, biceps, triceps, forearms, and finally, your neck and facial muscles.

When you finish correctly relaxing your body in the manner just described you will feel as though you are floating in space, and you won't be able to tell for sure the orientation of either your arms or legs. This is precisely how you feel when under deep hypnosis. And it is only logical, because mental visualization is a form of self-hypnosis.

As soon as you are fully relaxed, start to build an image in your mind of how you will look one year from now. You'll be able to "see" this image as though it is a film being projected against the insides of your eyelids.

Berry de Mey outside the Carlton Hotel, Cannes, France. ►

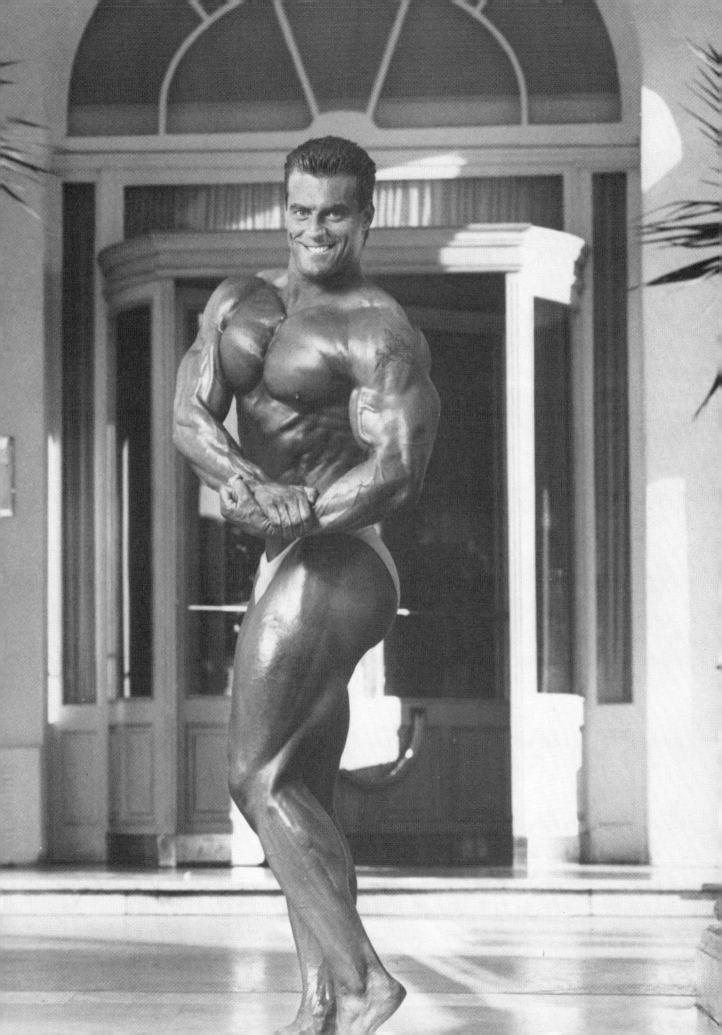

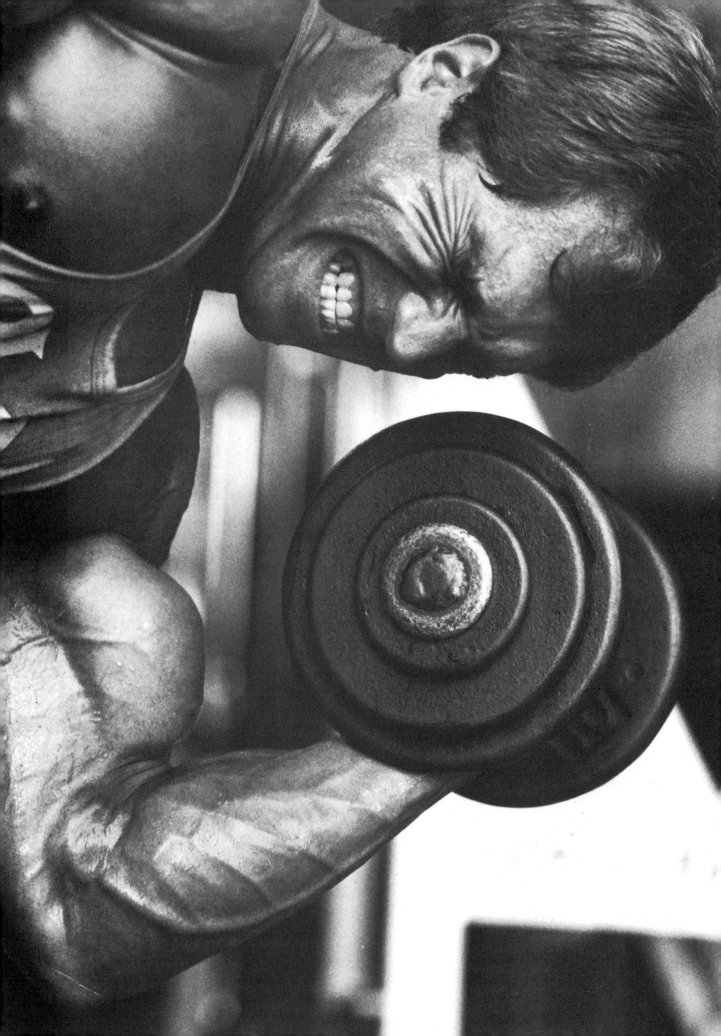

This visual image should show you in fantastically improved condition, but at the same time it should be a *realistic* image. As Tom Platz (IFBB Mr. Universe and a bodybuilder who has placed third in Mr. Olympia) wryly notes, "You can visualize playing pro basketball in the N.B.A. if you're only 5 feet tall, but it won't get you very far. Visualize some great improvements in your physique, but don't go overboard on the degree of improvement. Be sure you visualize physical qualities which are within your grasp."

As you work to generate this visual image, think about how 10 pounds of new muscle mass will look on your physique a year from now, how ripped up you'll be, how well you will have balanced your physical proportions and how much better you will present yourself onstage. This visual image should be so clear that you can see every ridge of muscle and valley of separation between muscles, as well as the thick, freewaylike tracery of veins over the muscles and just beneath your paper-thin skin.

At first it will be difficult to hold this hot new image of your physique for more than a few seconds before your mind skips off to another topic or problem. (We talked about this problem in chapter 3 when discussing the concept of mental concentration.) Whenever your mind skips off, *immediately* force it back on the image. With time and practice you will be able to maintain mental focus on your conjured-up image of your new

Dave Hawk does dumbbell preacher curls. ➤

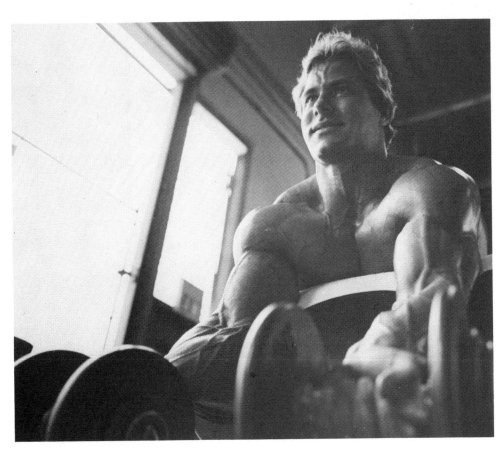

◄ Concentration curls: Gary Strydom.

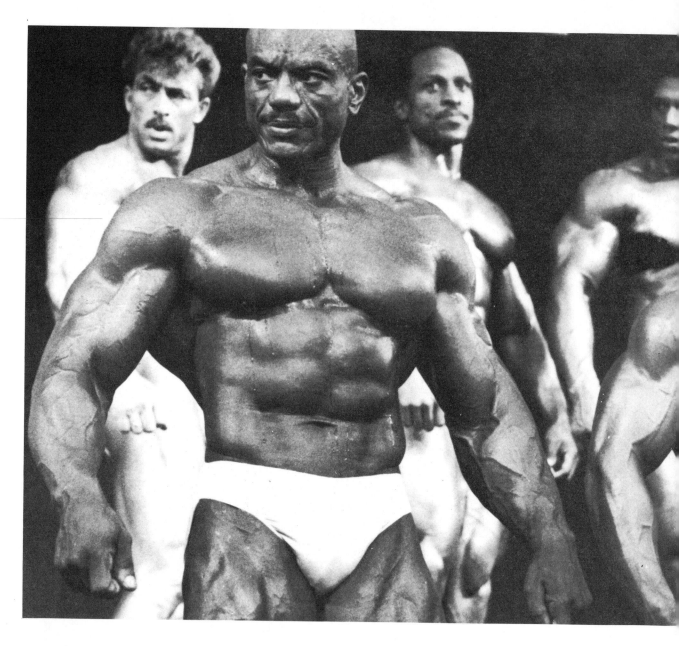

physique for increasingly longer periods of time. As soon as you can lie there in bed and savor your visualized image for 10–15 minutes at a time, you will have mastered the first step in using mental imagery to program your subconscious mind to assist you in your intense bodybuilding efforts throughout the day, throughout the year.

In the foregoing description of visualization, you have used the visualized image of sight. Usually that's as far as most bodybuilders and others take the visualization process. But psychologists have demonstrated that five-sense visualization is much more effective than normal, one-sense visualization. Once you've gotten visualized sight down pat, it's no problem at all—particularly not for a bodybuilder—to learn to visualize using the other four senses: hearing, touch, taste and olfactory ability.

Sensational Anja Langer, the sport's next superstar, tells about how she

▲ Front row, from left: Sergio Oliva, Samir Bannout, and Bill Grant at the 1984 Mr. Olympia in New York.

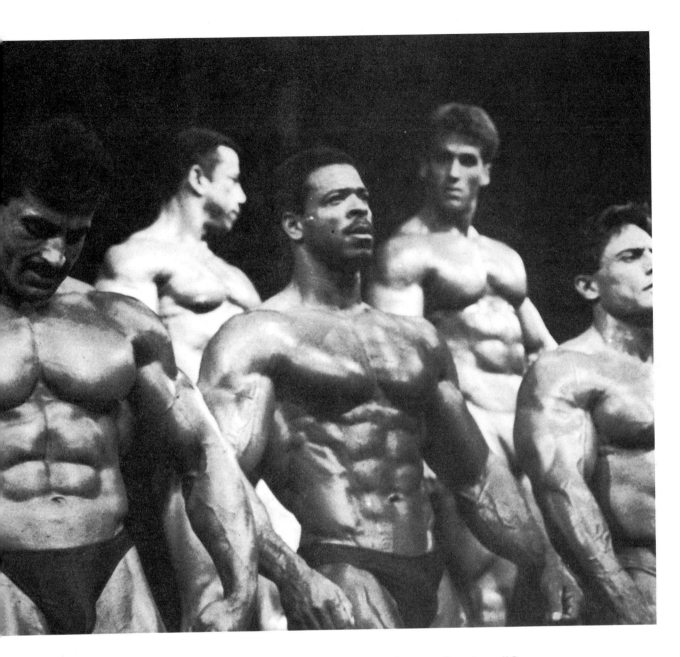

adds the sense of touch to her sight visualization: "Once you *see* your new body, try to project yourself into it, feeling every muscle contract and relax as you do chores around home, or get in a heavy bodybuilding workout. I *love* the powerful, mentally visualized feeling of being inside a sensational new physique. I often visualize myself dramatically improved and concurrently feel the muscles exerting against the weights as I pump up prior to going out onstage to compete. I can even look down at my feet and flexed calves as my legs propel me toward the middle of the stage for my prejudging. Every imagined movement I make accompanies an imagined feel of my powerful, high-quality new muscles contracting and extending, contracting and extending. It's a great feeling, because I *know* I will achieve that visualized image for my next Pro World Championship or Ms. Olympia!"

Let's give another terrific European, Holland's Berry de Mey (who has

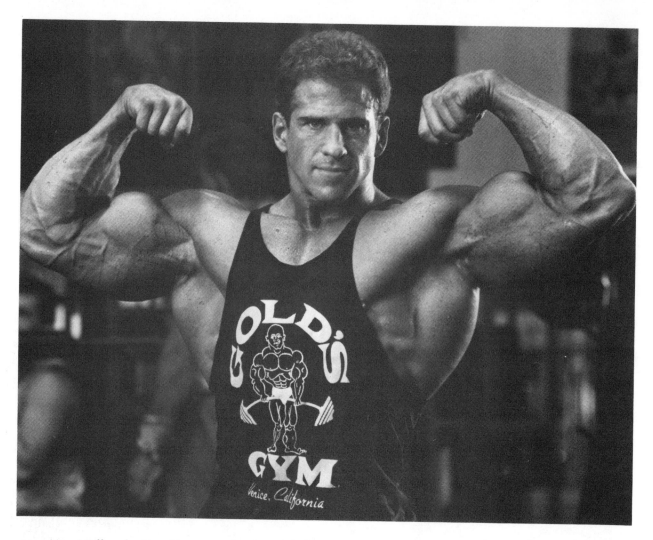

won Mr. Holland, Mr. Europe, the World Games Heavyweight Championship, and three times has been a Mr. Olympia finalist), a chance to tell how he adds the sense of smell to his visualized image of himself: "I most like to visualize myself either onstage at a competition or in the gym training, and in both cases I can imagine myself having a greatly improved physique, which I can actually feel when I pose onstage or do an imagined heavy set in the gym.

"Injecting my olfactory sense into my visualized image is a relatively simple matter. In my backstage warm-up room fantasy, I can smell the oil I rub into my skin to highlight my muscles. In the visualized gym setting, I can easily smell the tart, honest aroma of perspiration a hard workout brings out on all bodybuilders. It's also possible to mentally visualize the aroma of a precontest meal being prepared. But the diets of most of the top guys are so bland right before a contest that they usually have very little aroma, or at least nothing anyone might look forward to smelling."

Samir Bannout (Mr. Universe, Mr. World and Mr. Olympia) discusses how he injects sound into his visualized image: "I can think of two main situations in which sound is important to me, and I use each of these sounds

The immortal Dave ▶
Draper.

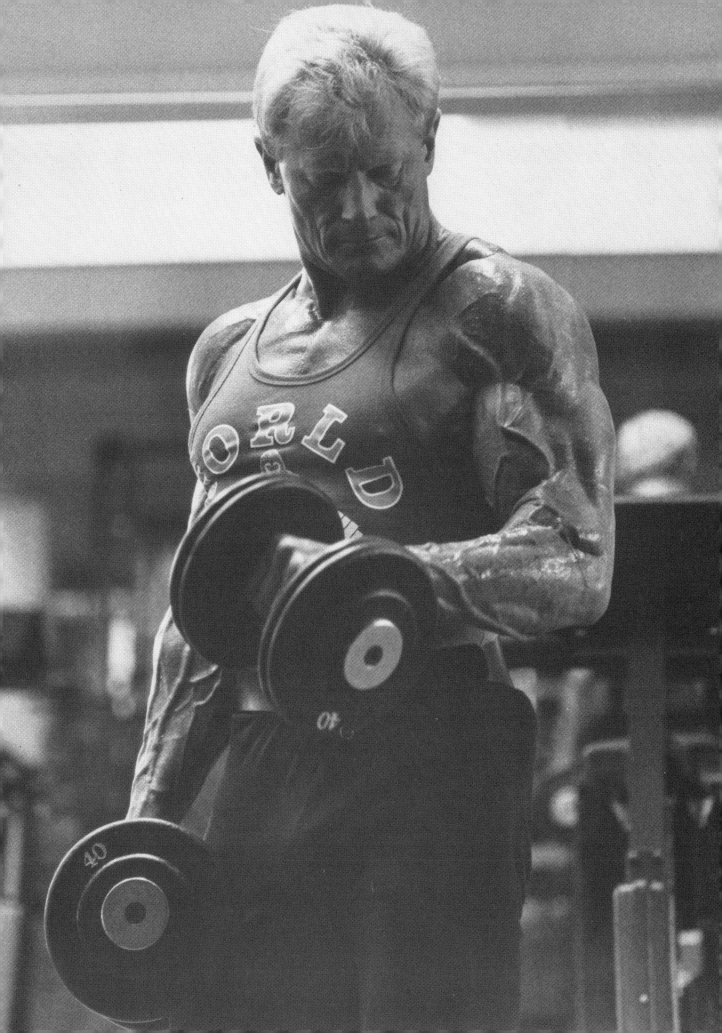

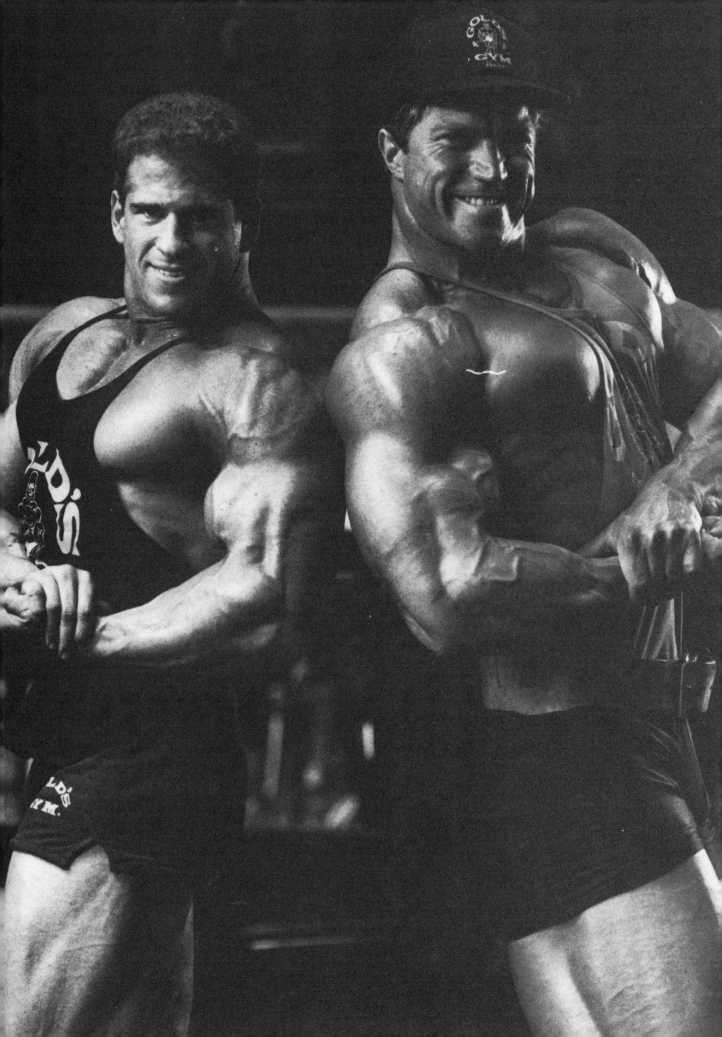

to improve my visualization practice. The first of these situations is the clang of the weights, the hot rock music and the general hubub at Gold's Gym in Venice, California, where I trained for my Mr. Olympia victory back in 1983. There's so much energy there in that gym when several of the sport's biggest stars are training at the same time. There's nothing like the deep-throated rattle of five 45-pound Olympic plates on each end of the bar as I perform a heavy set of squats, my muscles bulging with the effort.

"I remember all of these sounds and constantly reproduce them for my own inspiration and benefit when I'm practicing visualization each night. I see myself 6—8 pounds heavier and 10 percent more cut than the last time I competed, and I feel my huge new muscles lifting the weights in each exercise. Add in the sounds at Gold's Gym and you know why it was dubbed The Mecca of Bodybuilding.

"The second thing I can always remember and recreate in my mental imagery sessions in subsequent months is the roar of all my fans when I am going through my free-posing routine at an Olympia or other high-level pro show. My fans are the greatest, and I never let them down. So I also visualize myself in fantastic new physical condition walking onstage to the massed adulation of my fans. Their enthusiastic applause will always push me to continue improving and competing successfully for many more years."

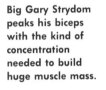

Big Gary Strydom peaks his biceps with the kind of concentration needed to build huge muscle mass.

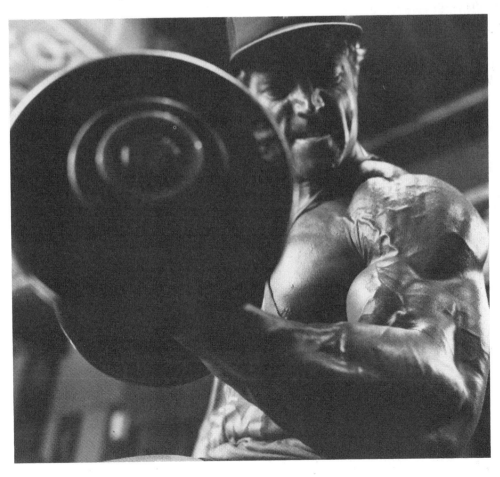

◄ Tom Terwilliger and Gary Strydom.

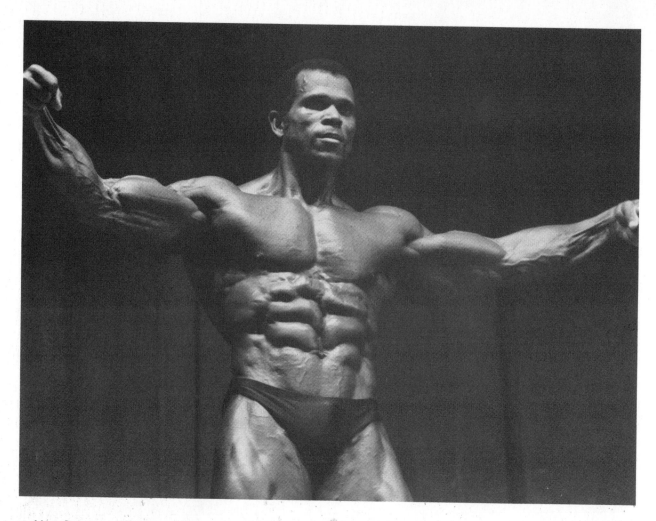

▲ The great Nubret
photographed in
Vienna in 1987.

Hot Suzanne Steurer (German and European Champion, plus a finalist in the IFBB World Championships) knows how to add the sense of taste to her visualized image of her great new physique: "I visualize myself with more massive muscles than ever before, and already with incredible muscular density and separation. With this physical image in mind, I imagine the taste of a dry, broiled, skinned chicken breast, or perhaps a nice dry, broiled piece of freshwater fish. Neither has much taste, but they do give me one more visualization variable to work with. I find it no problem to use all five senses in my visualization sessions. With only a bit of practice, no bodybuilder should have any problem doing so either."

At first it may take you 30 minutes to fully relax yourself and 30 minutes more to haphazardly work up a good visualized image. But with only three to four weeks of practice, you can be totally relaxed for a productive 10- to 15-minute visualization session in only about 10 minutes. And that's a very small price to pay for harnessing the power of your subconscious mind to help you build a world-class physique in record time!

Suzanne Steurer.  ➤

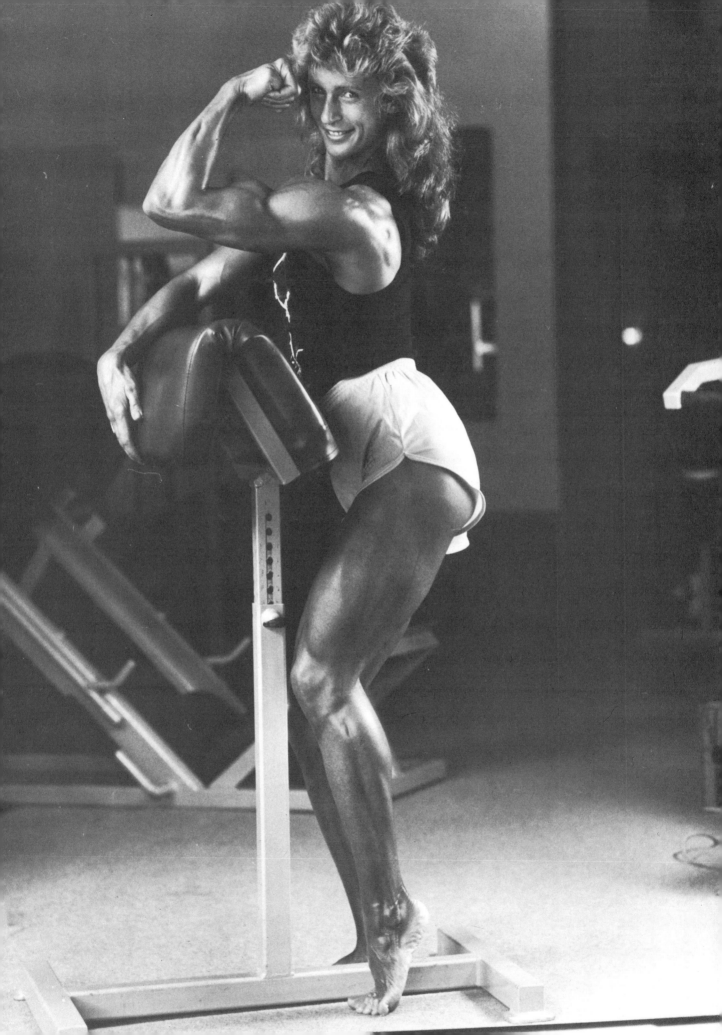

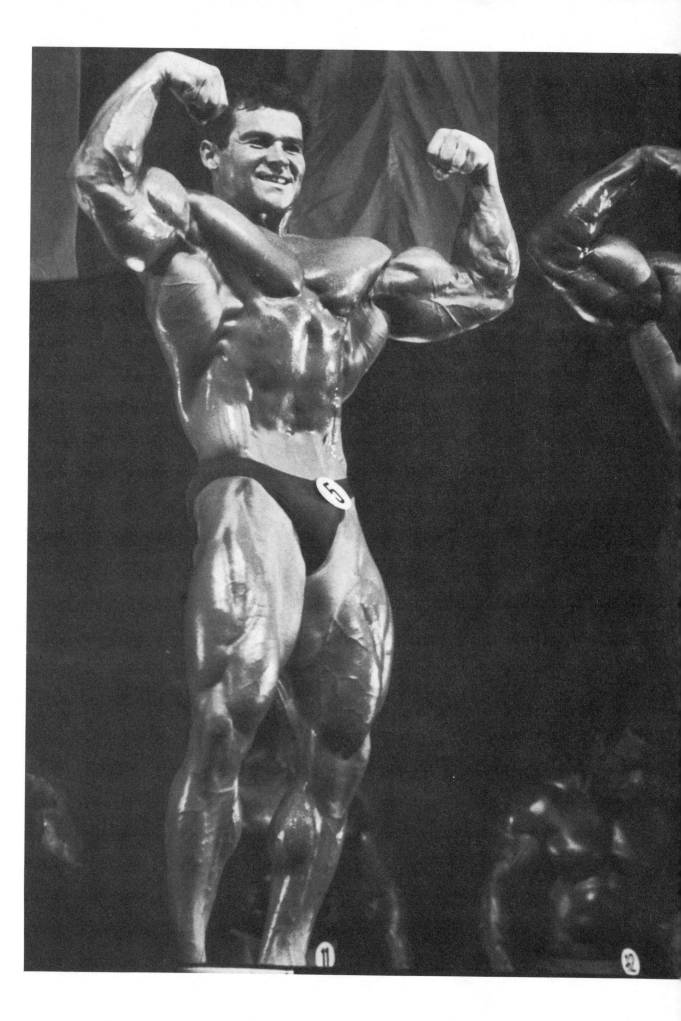

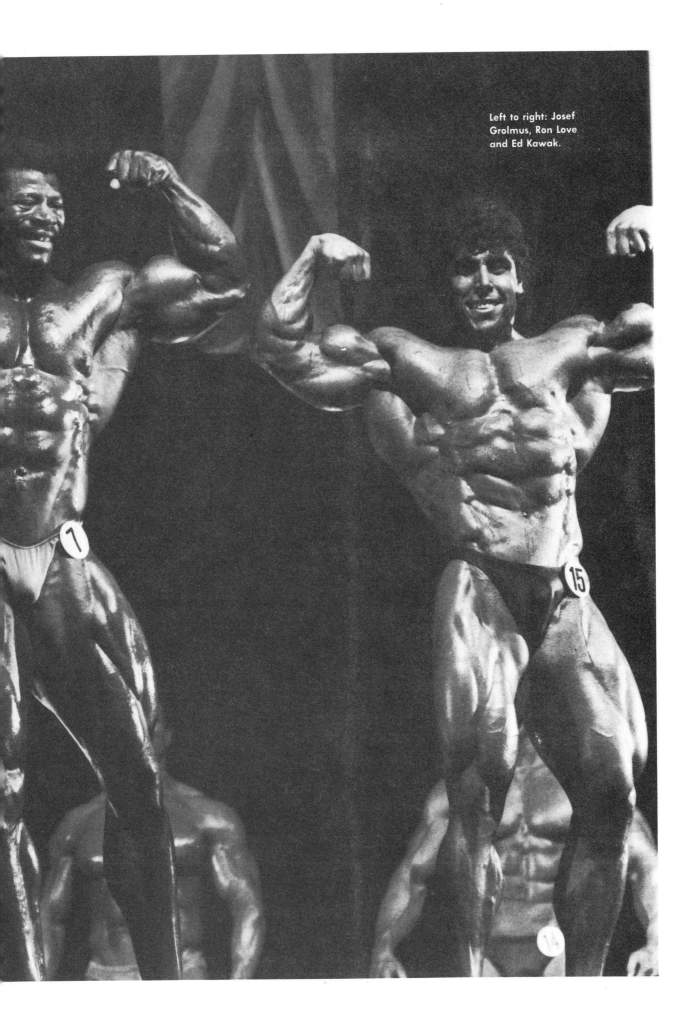

Left to right: Josef Grolmus, Ron Love and Ed Kawak.

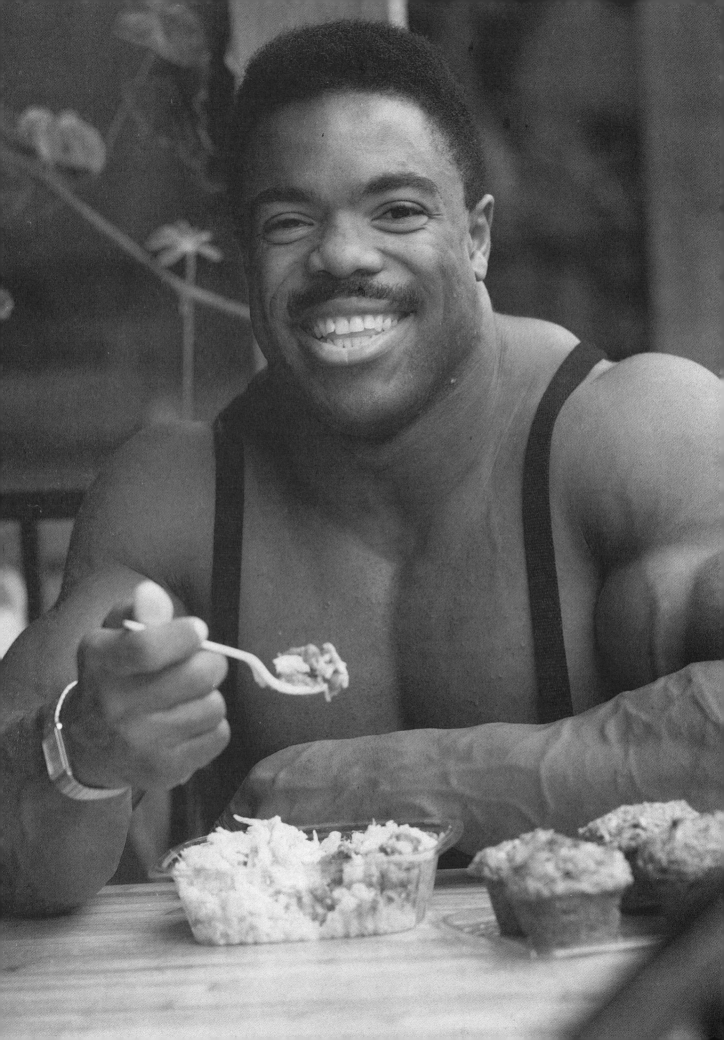

# 5

# Bodybuilding Nutrition

**R**egardless of how committed and well directed your mind might be and how intensely you pump iron in the gym, most of your efforts will go unrewarded if you fail to concurrently maintain an optimum bodybuilding nutrition plan. Indeed, virtually all bodybuilders believe strongly that training, mental approach and nutrition go hand in hand to develop great physiques.

Listen to what Lee Haney (second now only to Arnold Schwarzenegger in Mr. Olympia wins) has to say on these three vital subjects: "In my bodybuilding seminars around the world I characterize training, mental approach and proper nutrition as each being one leg of a tripod holding your physique aloft, out of the mud and away from the teeming masses who yearn to be built like you are.

"As long as you keep each of the three tripod legs strong, there will be no danger of you falling in the mud and being trampled. But if you begin to neglect any one of these tripod legs—whether it be training, mental approach or diet—the structure will begin to rock and roll. Finally, one of the legs will splinter, and you will fall to your bodybuilding death.

◄ Phil Hill.

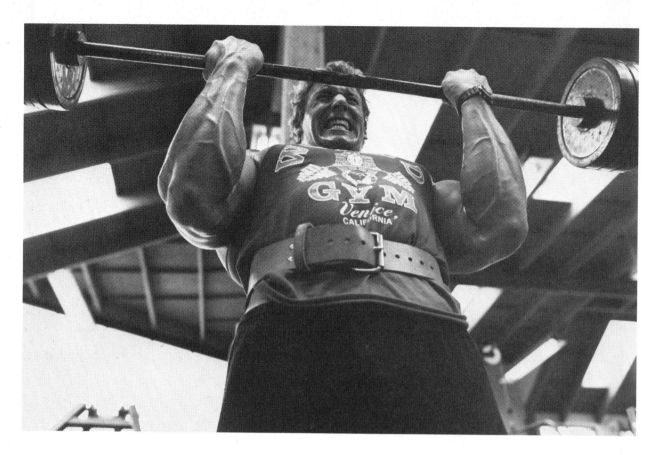

Standing barbell curl: Ralf Moeller.

"No doubt you feel that my tripod analogy is a little extreme. But it must be that way to convince bodybuilders of the great importance of high-intensity training, positive mental conditioning and optimum nutrition. Each leg of the tripod *must* be strong. Any one weak leg—no matter how strong the other two might be—and the tripod cannot stand erect!"

Anja Langer (Junior World Champion, European Champion and a great professional bodybuilder by the time she was only 20 years of age) says, "Assuming the correct mental approach is the glue which holds the entire bodybuilding process together, I feel training and diet are a fifty-fifty proposition in the off-season. And as a major competition approaches, the importance of correct diet increases, until it reaches a maximum level of about 80 percent of the battle just prior to a show. No serious body-builder—man or woman—can ever neglect diet and still expect to become a champion.

"During the final week before a Ms. Olympia competition I have come to believe diet is about 95 percent of the battle and training only 5 percent responsible for my onstage success. All of my training had its impact during the weeks and months leading up to a competition, and last-week training can do little to help or harm my appearance. But a wrong food here or there during that final precompetitive week can change my normally diamond-hard muscularity to both puffy and mushy. You must eat right to win!"

Luiz Freitas. ➤

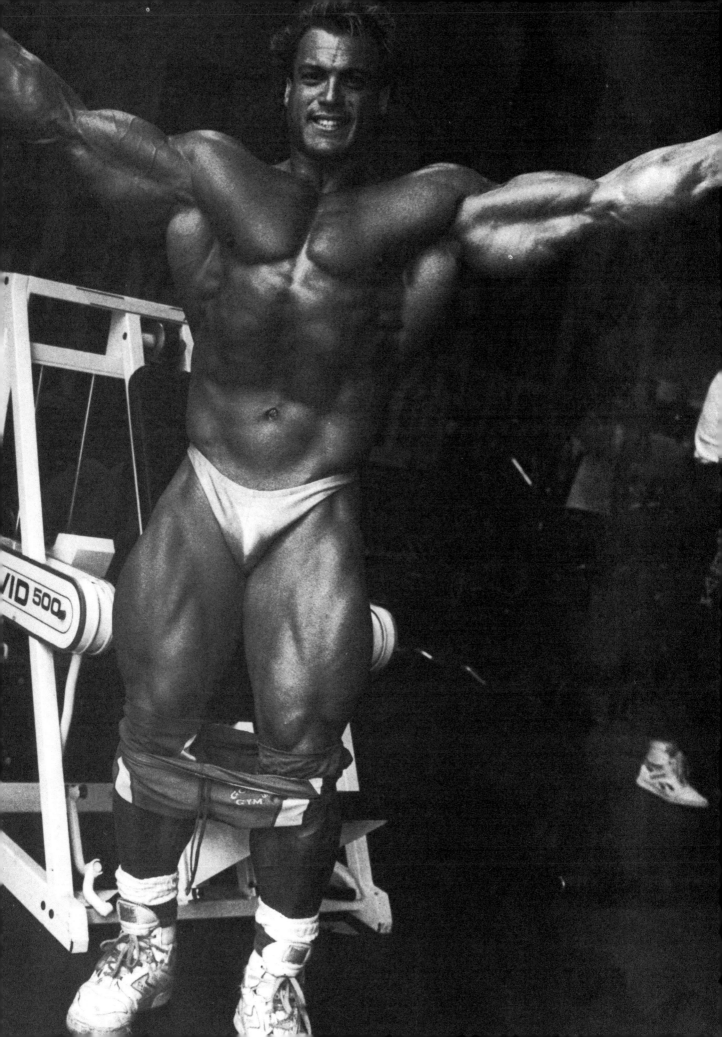

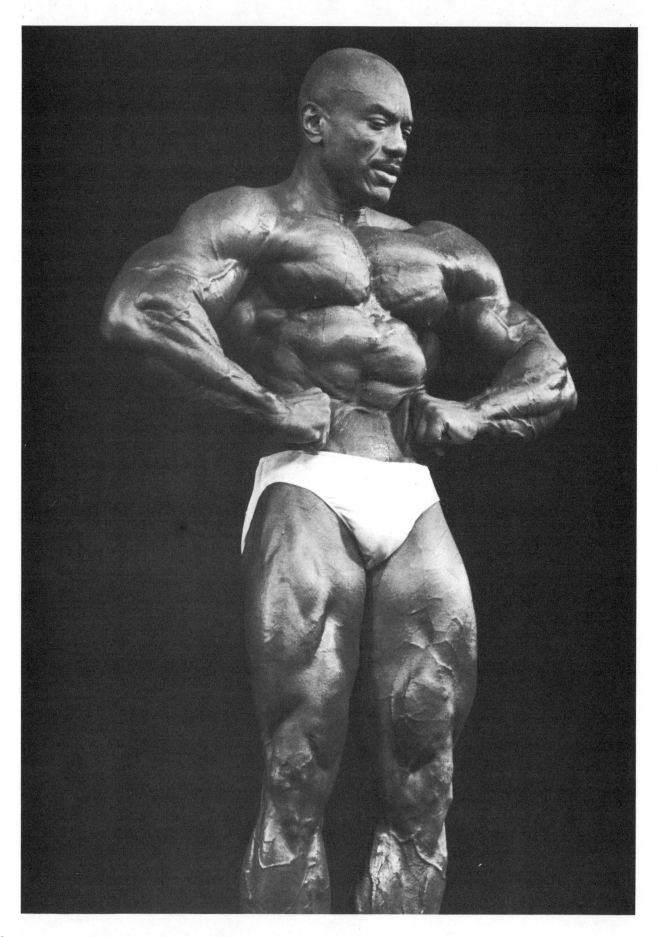

## Basic Food Elements

By and large, you can obtain virtually all of the food elements necessary for building huge, well-shaped and highly defined muscles. There are thousands of very good bodybuilders who use no food supplements at all. One good contemporary athlete who eschews the use of concentrated protein, amino acids, vitamins and minerals is massive Jim Quinn, who has won a host of amateur titles in Eastern America, including the Heavyweight and Overall Eastern USA Championships. You'll read a lot about Jim in future years, because he's a surefire National Champion and IFBB pro bodybuilder.

Stepping back ten to twelve years in time, Eddie Giuliani (who now manages Gold's World Gym in Venice, California) was one of the hottest bodybuilders when competing on the national—and occasionally international—level. In quick succession, he won Mr. California, Mr. Western America, and his height class in both the Mr. America and Mr. International shows. At the time he was still winning big, he told me about a very interesting experiment he conducted with food supplements.

◄ The Myth.

▼ Buddy bombing at Gold's: Luiz Freitas and Mike Christian.

"I had always been a mega-supplement user," Giuliani told me, "and credited much of my competitive bodybuilding success to my comprehensive use of the entire spectrum of food supplements. I was probably spending about $5000 per year on food supplements during that time period. I firmly

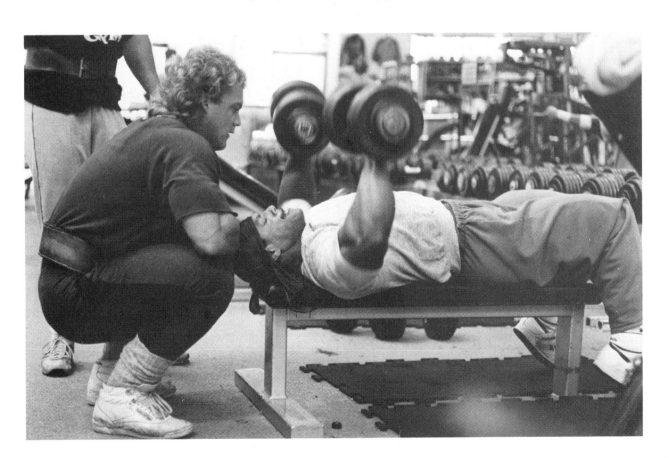

believed they kept me feeling great, and was convinced I could make no muscle gains whatsoever without virtually living on food supplements.

"Then just as an experiment I went one full year without taking a single food supplement, not even one capsule of multiple vitamins and minerals. The remainder of my diet was unchanged, except that I ate a bit more protein in the form of poultry, fish, raw and fertile eggs, and nonfat milk products. And do you know what happened? I felt every bit as good that year as I had felt when taking massive amounts of supplements, and I made some of my best gains in muscle mass that year.

"Today, I still train hard, I follow a basic, healthy, well-balanced diet with plenty of fresh foods and roughage. And I take one multipack of vitamins, minerals, enzymes and trace elements with each breakfast. My sense of well-being is better than it's ever been, I have more energy than ever before, and even though I'm no longer training for competition, my muscle mass and quality are superb. I wish I'd discovered this type of diet and moderate supplement program twenty years ago!"

There is considerable conjecture among champion and near-champion bodybuilders that massive amounts of food supplements are totally unnecessary. A respected East German track and field coach once joked, "American athletes must have the world's most expensive urine. They take huge dosages of vitamins and minerals, but the body can utilize only small amounts of each nutrient. The huge excess of unused nutrients are simply urinated from the body. What a waste!"

Then why do so many of the top guys in bodybuilding write articles about the huge dosages of inosine, B-15, or whatever else they might be taking, and endorse products for one of the supplements distributors? The answer is that good old America word, *money*. The top athletes are *paid* to promote use of high dosages of various elemental nutrients, thereby making lots more money for the supplements promoter/distributor.

Supplements distributors are laughing all the way to the bank with your money in their pockets if you are spending $500–$1000 per month on supplements (don't laugh, I know many bodybuilders who virtually live on supplements). You can easily supplement your diet with all of the food concentrates you would require to win Mr. or Ms. Olympia for less than $100 per month. Let me tell you how.

### Protein and Amino Acids

You'll see an article on either protein or amino acid supplements in virtually every issue of each bodybuilding magazine owned by one food supplements distributor. You are bombarded with data about how human muscle tissue is comprised of twenty-two building blocks called amino acids, all but eight of which can be manufactured within your body. These eight

Graham McGregor ➤ holds back the animal in Mike Quinn.

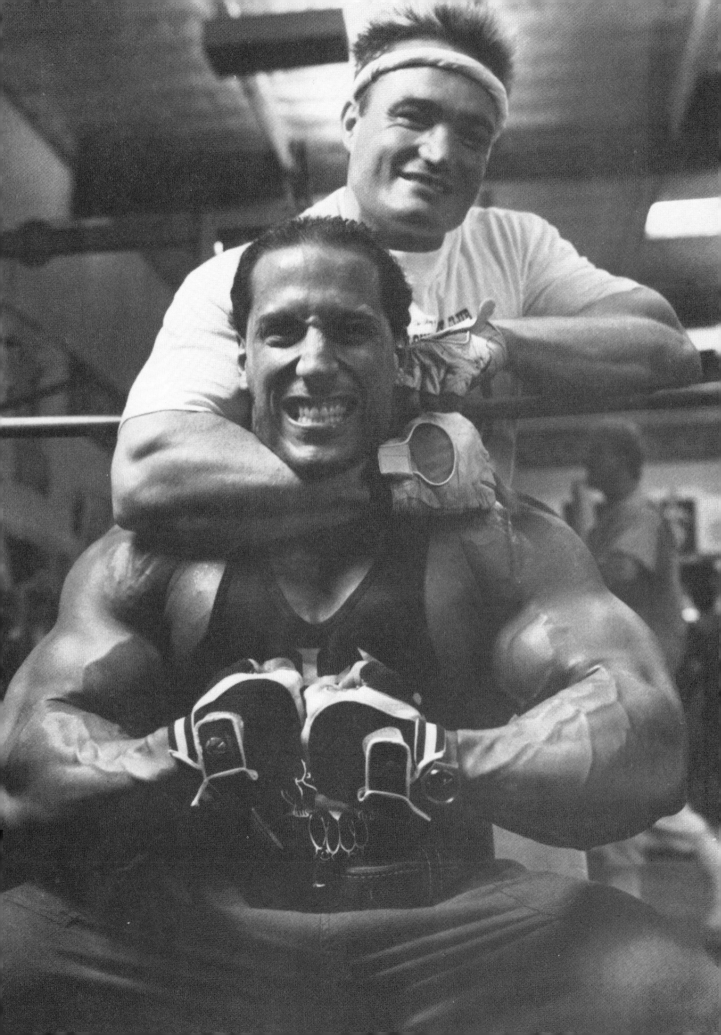

essential amino acids must be supplied by your daily diet, or your muscles can't grow. That's why you need to consume 3–4 pounds of milk-and-egg protein powder and 400–500 free-form amino acid capsules per month, so they say.

As you study Zen, you will discover the Zen way is always simple, logical, realistic and to the point. The Zen approach to bodybuilding could never insist you take all of these protein concentrates and amino acid capsules. Your body can get along just fine without them.

Most vegetable protein is incomplete, which means it is either missing—or has very low amounts of—one or more of the eight essential amino acids. But all you need to complete protein from vegetable sources, thereby making it suitable for use in building muscle tissue, is to eat the vegetable protein with a small amount of animal protein, particularly eggs or milk.

In many cases, you can complete the protein in one vegetable food by eating it in the same meal as one other selected vegetable food. For example, you can combine any legume (beans, peas, peanuts, etc.) with any grain, seed or nut. The protein in each element alone is incomplete, but when they are combined together, each completes the protein count of the other food.

Supplements distributors constantly run articles in their magazines "explaining" why bodybuilders need 200–300 grams of protein per day to build muscle mass. I've personally known over 100 top bodybuilders who ate 300+ grams of protein daily for years. I know one who consumes 80 to 100 eggs per day!

The FDA (United States Food and Drug Administration) has run hundreds of experiments to determine protein requirements for children and adults of both sexes, plus for lactating women. It has established an AMDR (Adult Minimum Daily Requirement) for protein of one gram per kilogram (2.2 pounds) of body weight. The AMDR goes upward a bit—but only a bit—for lactating women, but the FDA has concluded that physical activity does *not* increase the AMDR level.

What this means is that a 198-pound man (90 kilograms) can gain muscle mass quite readily on 90 grams of good-quality protein. And many very good bodybuilders have maintained—even improved—their outstanding physiques on even less protein. Mike Mentzer (Mr. America, Mr. Universe and Heavyweight Mr. Olympia) weighed 215 pounds when he won his first professional competition, and he rarely consumed more than 60 grams of protein per day. Venerable Bill Pearl (winner of four NABBA Mr. Universe titles) carries 240 pounds of solid muscle mass at 50 years of age, and he hasn't eaten more than 70–75 grams of protein per day for many years. Pearl is also a lacto-vegetarian, and doesn't eat flesh foods.

So where does this leave you? I suggest eating four times per day at

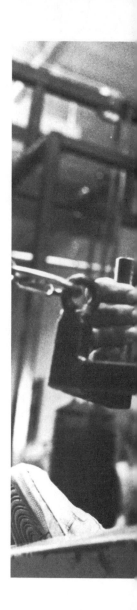

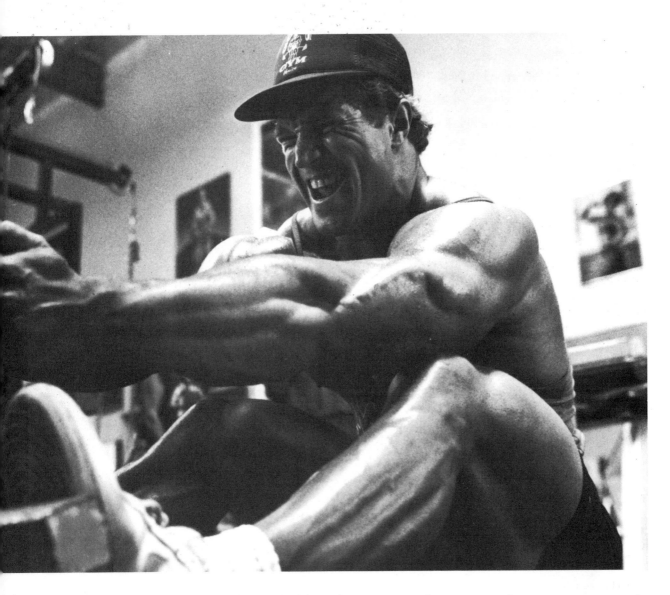

▲ Seated low-pulley rowing is the favorite back exercise of almost every bodybuilder.

intervals of 3–3½ hours between meals. Be sure there is some animal-source protein in each of your meals. Here's an example of such a diet for one day:

*Meal 1*—Six-egg omelette with cheese and mushrooms; fruit; 1-2 slices of whole-grain toast; milk; supplements multipack

*Meal 2*—Tuna salad with a minimum of low-cal dressing; 1–2 baked potatoes (dry); 1–2 green vegetables or a large, fresh, green salad; iced tea or coffee or milk

*Meal 3*—Large Caesar salad with plenty of greens, diced cold meat and cheese, walnuts, sunflower seeds, hardboiled eggs and any other ingredient you prefer; iced tea or milk

*Meal 4*—Broiled steak; rice; 1–2 green/yellow vegetables; 1–2 slices of toasted whole-grain bread; sorbet or fresh fruit for dessert; coffee or milk

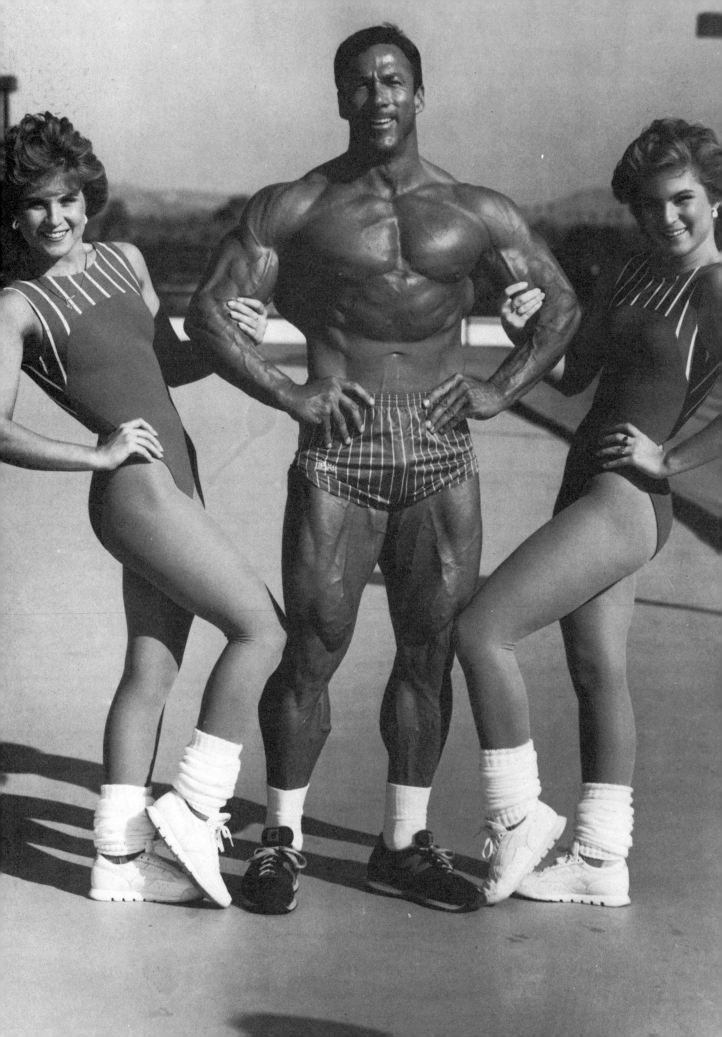

If you finally conclude that you need to take a protein supplement, purchase only a milk-and-egg powder, because milk and eggs are of very high biological quality and easily digested and assimilated into muscle tissue. Take a protein shake *only between meals* rather than with meals. If you take only one shake per day, consume it 30 minutes before training. If you wish a second shake, drink it about 45 minutes before going to bed and falling asleep each night.

Following is a recipe for a delicious protein shake which can be mixed in a variable-speed blender:

- 8–10 ounces of low-fat milk (raw milk is best)
- ½ cup of shaved ice (optional)
- 1½–2 tablespoons of milk-and-egg protein powder
- 1–2 pieces of fresh, soft fruit (peaches, bananas, strawberries and blueberries are all great)

Put in the milk and start the blender up at a slow speed. Add ice, if desired, and blend at a high speed for about 30 seconds. Slow the blender and slowly sift in the protein powder. Finally, add the fruit and gradually increase blender speed until all fruit has been chopped fine and everything is well mixed. For an occasional taste treat, try blending vanilla ice cream, finely chopped dates, milk and protein powder.

These protein shakes taste best poured right from the blender into a frosted glass, but they can also be stored for up to 24 hours in a thermos jug and shaken up by hand to remix settled ingredients before drinking the concoction. This way you can take a protein drink with you to school or work.

At the beginning of this section I mentioned free-form amino acid capsules. If you've priced them at a health food store or through ads in muscle magazines, you already know they are phenomenally expensive. It is also my highly experienced belief that free-form aminos are of value to competitive bodybuilders at the highest levels of the sport. But for most readers of this book, aminos are a colossal waste of money.

## Vitamins, Minerals and Enzymes

Since about 1980, multipacks of vitamins, minerals, enzymes and trace elements have been available to bodybuilders. Prior to that you would have had to carry around individual bottles of each supplement you wanted to take, open each one to remove a couple of tablets or capsules, then swallow all of them. Compared to tearing open a cellophane envelope prefilled with several capsules and tablets which have been scientifically selected to meet a bodybuilder's supplemental nutrition needs, going into

◄ Boyer Coe and friends.

one bottle after another now seems like something an iron-pumping trog-lodyte might do.

One multipack per day will meet the needs of any hard-training body-builder for vitamins, minerals, trace elements and enzymes. It should always be taken *with* a meal—preferably with breakfast—in order to foster op-timum assimilation of the nutrients in the capsules and tablets of the mul-tipack.

Shopping for multipacks (and all other food supplements) can be a little tricky until you have learned to read the labels on the boxes in which multipacks come. First be sure that the minerals contained in each packet are protein chelated; if not, they are virtually useless. Then compare all of the nutrient potencies from one brand of multipack to all of the others. Be careful that you compare potencies for *one* packet of each brand. A few unscrupulous supplements distributors give potencies for two or three packets, and list that fact somewhere on the box in type so small that a mouse wearing bifocals couldn't read it.

Several brands of multipacks now offer "timed-release" vitamins and minerals. In timed-release tablets, layers of the supplement nutrient are alternated with layers of some relatively inert substance (cornstarch is frequently used for the timed-release barrier coatings).

When you swallow a timed-release vitamin C tablet, for example, the vitamin is released each time the inert coating has been digested. And once that layer of vitamin C has been exhausted, the stomach's digestive acids must again eat through the inert layer before more vitamin C is released.

Timed-release coatings on water-soluble vitamins (B complex and C, mainly) are very valuable. Water-soluble vitamins are quickly passed out of your body through your urinary tract when large dosages of B or C are taken only once or twice a day. With timed-release B complex and C, small amounts are released many times per day, and these small amounts of the water-soluble nutrients are used much more completely and efficiently than vitamins which are not time released.

The father of timed-release medicines and food supplements was a Sicilian biochemist named Dr. Anthony Pescetti. He could actually put up to forty coatings on each tablet, although the norm in the food supplement industry is about ten to twelve coatings. Dr. Carlin Venus, who owns the Super Spectrim supplement company is using Pescetti's process, and he has a wonderful 12-hour timed-release vitamin-mineral tablet which I personally use to maintain good health and keep my energy levels high. If you'd like information about this supplement, write to Dr. Venus at 2666 Calle Man-zano, Thousand Oaks, CA 91360. If you want to save some time in ob-taining the information you are requesting, the telephone number there is 805-492-0455.

Bill Pearl. ➤

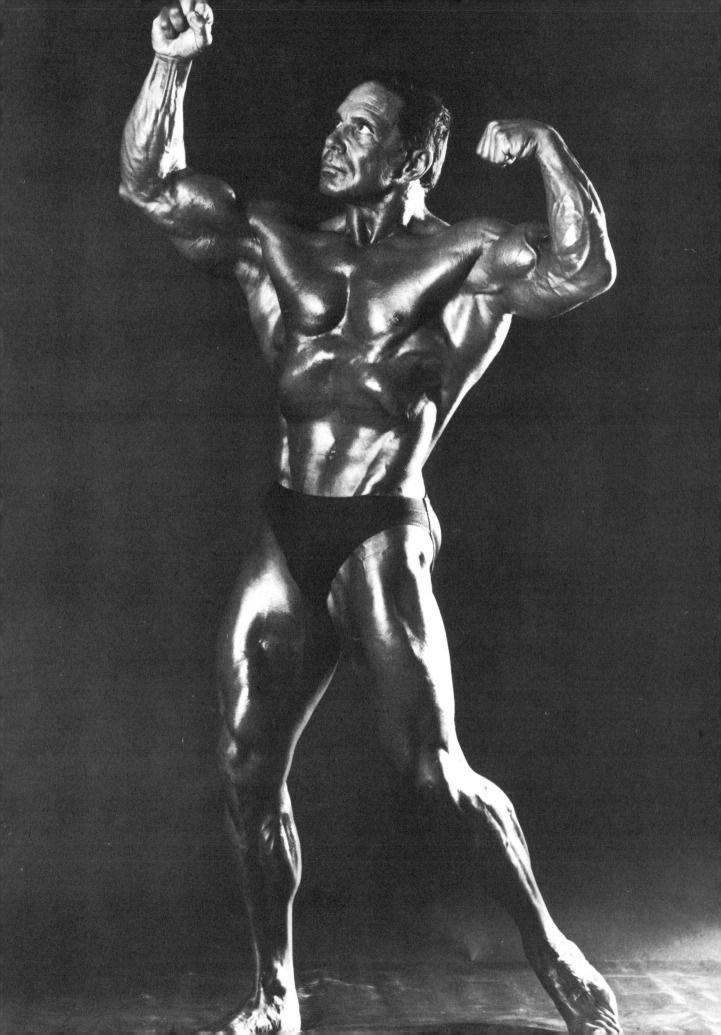

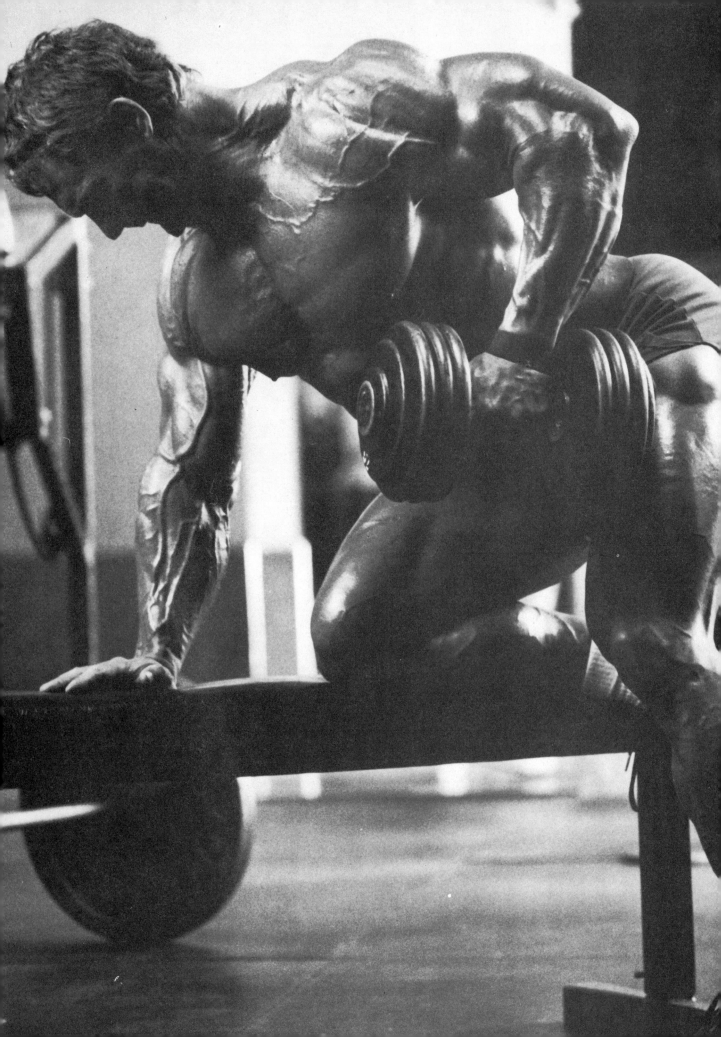

It is probable that this timed-release multiple vitamin-mineral tablet is an even more efficient means of supplementing your diet, and it is worth looking into the subject. A couple of top bodybuilders who take Dr. Venus's supplements are Jeff King (Mr. America, Mr. Universe) and Vincent Comerford (Mr. USA and NPC National Middleweight Champion).

Getting back to purchasing multipacks, compare all of the potencies of all nutrients available in various packets—checking for mineral chelation and timed-release factors—then compare the best three or four brands for cost effectiveness. Only then should you make a purchase. If you have trouble deciding which packets to buy, try writing everything down in a notebook, sleeping on it, and then making your decision in the morning. Usually, this will allow your subconscious mind sufficient time to make the decision for you.

Should you decide to invest in a couple of individual vitamin supplements to complement your multipacks, vitamin B complex and vitamin C are the most important to a hard-training bodybuilder. Again, they should be either time released, or taken every couple of hours throughout the day. The various B-complex vitamins help considerably to increase lean muscle tissue, while C is a natural detoxifying agent that cleans various pollutants and other poisons from your system.

At a supermarket or drugstore you can purchase an inexpensive, high-potency B-complex capsule (there should be at least 50 mg. of each B vitamin in the formulation). You can also buy vitamin C at a supermarket or pharmacy. It's much less expensive than B complex. Each of these supplements should be taken with meals. But never take B complex closer than 3–4 hours before going to bed; it can irritate your stomach lining and cause temporary insomnia.

### Useless Food Supplements

While they do work to a small degree, there are four individual food supplements that are virtually worthless to bodybuilders, despite grand claims for some of them from promoters who stress how valuable these nutrients are to hard-training athletes. The worthless supplements—you should avoid wasting hard-earned money on them—are dolomite, desiccated liver, kelp tablets, and capsules or tablets (even entire multipacks) which are claimed to have in them "anabolic" nutritional factors.

Dolomite is a highly touted source of calcium and magnesium. Indeed, there is plenty of calcium and magnesium in dolomite, but it is not chelated and therefore can't be used by the human body to satisfy nutritional needs. Dolomite is actually ground-up marble (marble of the kind Michelangelo used to carve his famous statues, David and the Pietà) which is bound together and compressed into a tablet. Dolomite is so useless that I know

◀ One-arm rows: Scott Wilson.

many bodybuilders who have seen complete, undigested tablets of the rock that have come through the entire digestive system and were eliminated in the stool.

Desiccated liver is touted as a wonderful food for producing superhuman workout endurance, and many young bodybuilders swallow up to 100 tablets per day. The supplements promotors base these claims on a lab experiment in which three groups of lab rats were fed different diets. Group One ate the normal lab-rat diet, Group Two that diet plus synthetic vitamins, and Group Three ate the normal lab-rat diet plus all of the desiccated liver they desired to consume.

After several weeks on the various diets, each group was cast into a separate drum of water, where each rat was forced to swim or drown. Group One rats swam about 15 minutes on an average before drowning, and Group Two rats held out only a couple of minutes longer. The Group Three rats, however, swam three to four times longer than any of the other rats, and two of Group Three rats were still swimming vigorously when the experiment was terminated after 2 hours. I think those two rats have been trading off lowering the record for the swim across the English Channel ever since the experiment.

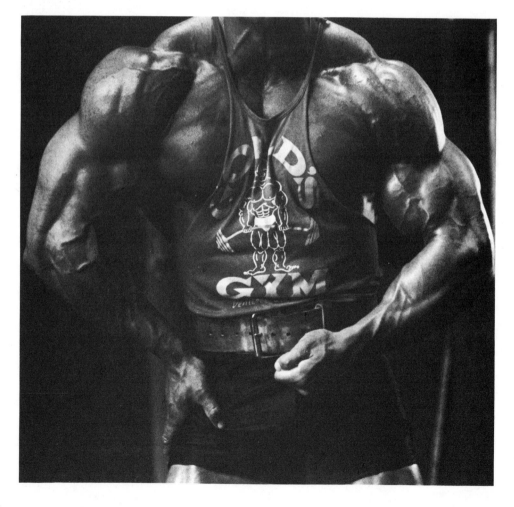

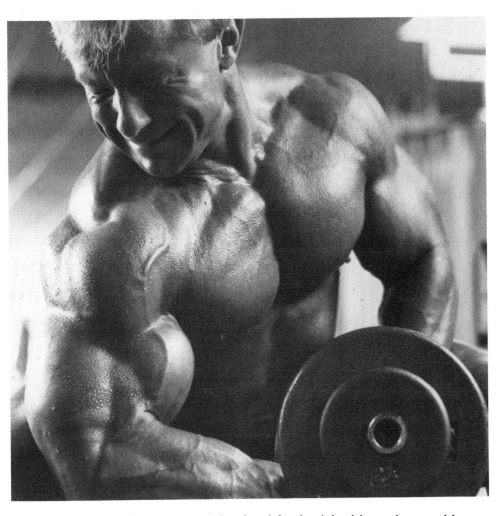

Vince Comerford. ➤

So, desiccated liver is a wonder food for bodybuilders who need better endurance, right? No says Michael Walczak, M.D., a leading bodybuilding nutritionist practicing in Van Nuys, California. "A normal lab-rat diet is very low in protein, while desiccated liver contains about 70 percent protein. The great difference in amount of protein intake by each lab-rat group made the difference, not some secret energy ingredient."

Dr. Walczak is also down on kelp tablets: "Scores of bodybuilders take handfuls of kelp tablets close to a competition, believing that the iodine in kelp will speed up their thyroids, enhance metabolism, making it easier to get ripped up. But iodine actually *lowers* the BMR. Physicians administer to hyperthyroid patients Lugol's solution—a suspension of iodine in water—to slow down metabolic rates."

Kelp does have a wealth of trace elements and should be taken during the off-season for those nutrients, but only in small quantities. Kelp is also very high in sodium, which could be death to peak muscularity if taken during the week leading up to a competition.

With the dramatic move toward natural (drug-free) bodybuilding in recent years, there has been a proliferation of nutritional supplements that contain natural anabolic nutritional factors. None of these supplements does for a bodybuilder what the promoters claim. Other claims are merely laughable, such as for orchic, which is only dried bulls' testicles. Moo to you, too, Molly!

Certain research does indicate that elements like arginine and ornithine (two amino acids), and several other nutritional elements, have an anabolic effect on the body. What you're not told is that the lab rats that showed increased STH (somatotrophic hormone, or human growth hormone) on arginine and ornithine, were taking 10,000 times as much per day as you get in your handy little megaanabolic packet. My advice is to spend your money on good food, train hard and heavy and get plenty of rest. You'll grow much faster that way than if you waste money on the megawhatever supplements.

## Weight-Loss Diet

"Simply losing weight is rather easy," notes gorgeous Anja Langer. "The trick is to lose body fat while maintaining muscle mass at its existing level. But if you allow yourself sufficient time—about one month per 3–4 pounds for women and a month per 5–6 pounds for men—you can burn off any excess body fat which is ruining the aesthetic appeal of your physique. And you will accomplish this task through a combination of low-fat dieting and aerobic exercise.

"Fat is a very concentrated form of calories, more than twice as rich in calories than either protein or carbohydrate of the same measure. In order to reduce calories and burn off excess body fat stores, you must limit— often down to almost zero—all dietary fat consumption. Foods high in fat include all oils, butter, full-fat milk and milk products, cream, egg yolks, pork, bacon, beef, poultry skin, avocados, corn, seeds and nuts. So you should avoid all of these foods when dieting to lose body fat. And at the same time you must keep your intake of protein and carbohydrate foods high, particularly the amount of complex carbohydrates you consume. You can't eat too much complex carbohydrate food."

Following is a one-day meal plan recommended by Anja Langer for body fat loss (this is a women's diet; men should eat proportionately more):

*Breakfast*—Whole-grain cereal with nonfat milk; 3–4 egg whites; piece of fruit; coffee; supplements

*Lunch*—Broiled fish; dry baked potato; green salad, with vinegar and lemon juice for dressing; one apple; iced tea

*Dinner*—Broiled white chicken meat (skin removed prior to cooking); brown rice; one green vegetable; perhaps also one yellow vegetable; one apple; icewater

Tom Terwilliger and Gary Strydom "flex it" for the camera of Chris Lund. ➤

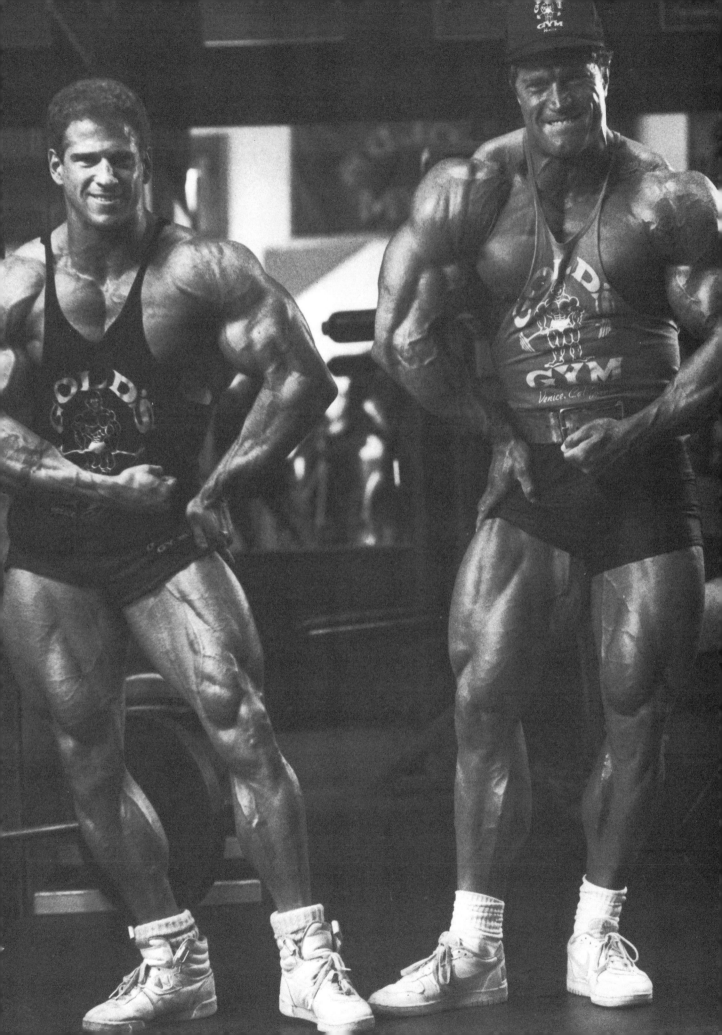

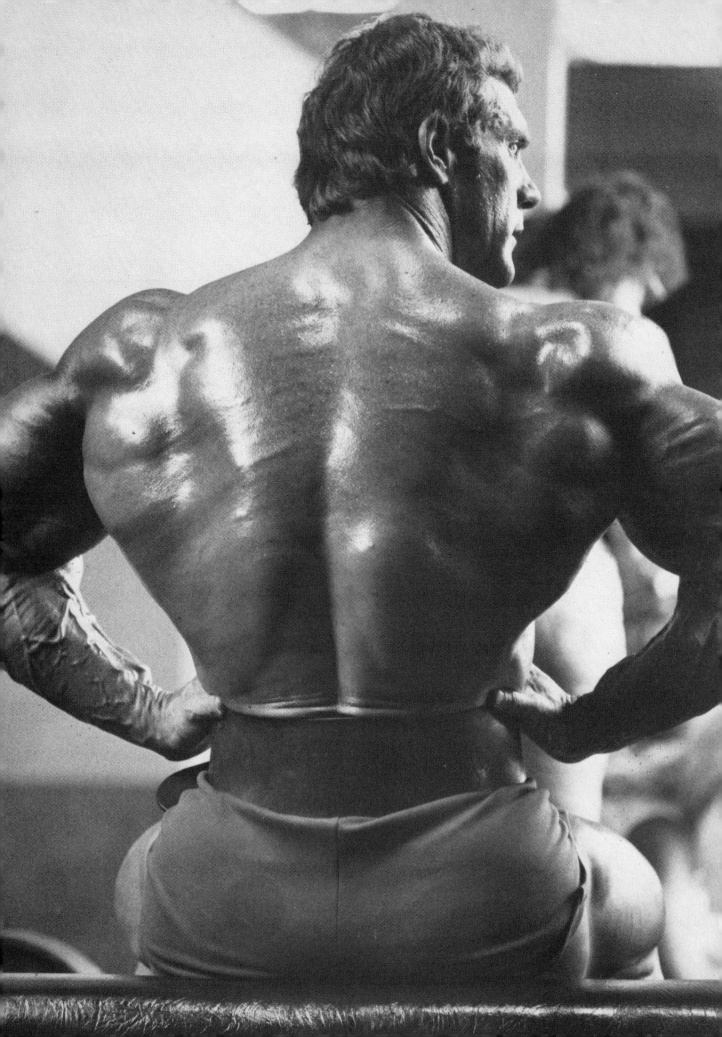

"You should break into this diet rather slowly," Anja advises, "gradually eliminating foods on your prohibited list. When you can see your muscle definition begin to improve from day to day—but you still have sufficient energy to train hard—you know instinctively that you are eating the correct number of calories."

Massive Scott Wilson (Pro Mr. America, Pro Mr. International and an IFBB Pro Grand Prix Champion) used to have trouble getting ripped up for a show, but now has his problem totally under control. "I used to eat as few as 1500 calories per day, but couldn't get off the excess body fat," he exclaims. "I was even riding a stationary cycle 2 or 3 hours per day and couldn't get cut. The problem was that I wasn't eating frequently enough—usually only two or three times per day—and that was slowing down my metabolism to the point where I couldn't burn off excess fat.

"Eating frequently has improved my metabolism so much that I can now get ripped up on 3000 calories per day, twice what I used to consume when I couldn't get cut to save my life. But I now eat small portions eight or nine times per day, roughly at 2-hour intervals. This way my muscle mass is high, and my body fat low despite having discontinued cycling. If your metabolism is slow, eat more often, not less often."

Diet should be combined with aerobic training in most cases, however. The anaerobic work of bodybuilding training takes its energy from glycogen stored in the muscles and liver, and hence burns very little fat. Aerobic training—long-lasting, low-intensity work—primarily burns stored body fat, so it's best for losing fat weight while retaining muscle mass.

The most popular forms of aerobic activity among top bodybuilders are stationary cycling, road cycling, running, fast walking, stair climbing, swimming and aerobic dance classes. When attempting to lose excess stored body fat, you should do at least one 30-minute aerobic workout each day, preferably at least 4–5 hours apart from your weight session. Or better yet, two 30-minute aerobic sessions each day should be taken, one in the morning and the other later in the day.

### Weight-Gain Diet

The object of a weight-gain diet is to eat to increase muscle mass while limiting any excess increase in body fat. The object is *not* to pig out on ice cream and other junk food, sleep half of the day, take a desultory workout and end up looking porcine at best.

I can't think of a better bodybuilder to discuss weight gain than hulking Lou Ferrigno (who won two IFBB Mr. Universe titles prior to taking up acting). With a height of 6 feet 5 inches, Louie reached a super-hard contest body weight of 275 pounds, ultimately taking runner-up position in the Mr. Olympia, second only to Arnold Schwarzenegger. And all of

*◀ The magnificent back of Scott Wilson.*

this from a kid who started out weighing only about 150 pounds.

"The crucial aspect of a weight-gain diet," Ferrigno explains, "is its emphasis on muscle-building protein content. The human stomach can only digest about 25 grams of protein per meal, and even less than that when the stomach has been crammed with protein foods. That just makes the protein digestion process more inefficient than it already is, so bodybuilders seeking to gain weight should limit protein intake at each meal to about 25 grams.

"At a rate of three meals per day, however, your digestive system would only process and make ready for assimilation into muscle a total of 75 grams of protein. So in order to increase the amount of protein digested each day, weight-gaining bodybuilders usually eat six small meals per day—at intervals of 2½–3 hours—rather than the usual two or three larger feasts most people eat each day. Six protein-rich meals will double the amount of protein digested in comparison to only three meals.

"The best protein foods come from animal sources. They include beef, poultry, fish, other seafood, eggs, milk and milk products, and they should be consumed at every meal at a rate of 25 total grams of protein. It's also a good practice to rotate protein foods from meal to meal—beef one meal, eggs the next, shellfish the third one, and so forth throughout the day.

"You will take in a moderate amount of fat when eating animal-protein foods, but you needn't worry about that when you are training consistently hard. With hard, heavy workouts, your metabolism will go up and you might feel hungry more frequently. As long as you satisfy those hunger pangs with good protein foods—not rich, gourmet ice cream—go ahead and eat whenever you are hungry, even if it is more than six times per day.

"The protein in each meal should be complemented with large servings of complex carbohydrate foods, which give you the energy to blast through even the heaviest workouts. My personal favorite complex carb foods are pasta, potatoes, rice, beans and fruit. But you can also eat any type of tuber, grain, lentil, seed or nut to fulfill your requirement for energy-releasing complex carbohydrate foods."

In addition to eating correctly, Louie suggests hard, heavy, basic workouts to help increase muscle mass. You will find these precise training programs in the next chapter. With Ferrigno's weight-gain diet and these workouts, you will pile on muscle faster and more easily than you could ever have dreamed possible, whether or not you are taking growth drugs!

Mike Mentzer. ➤

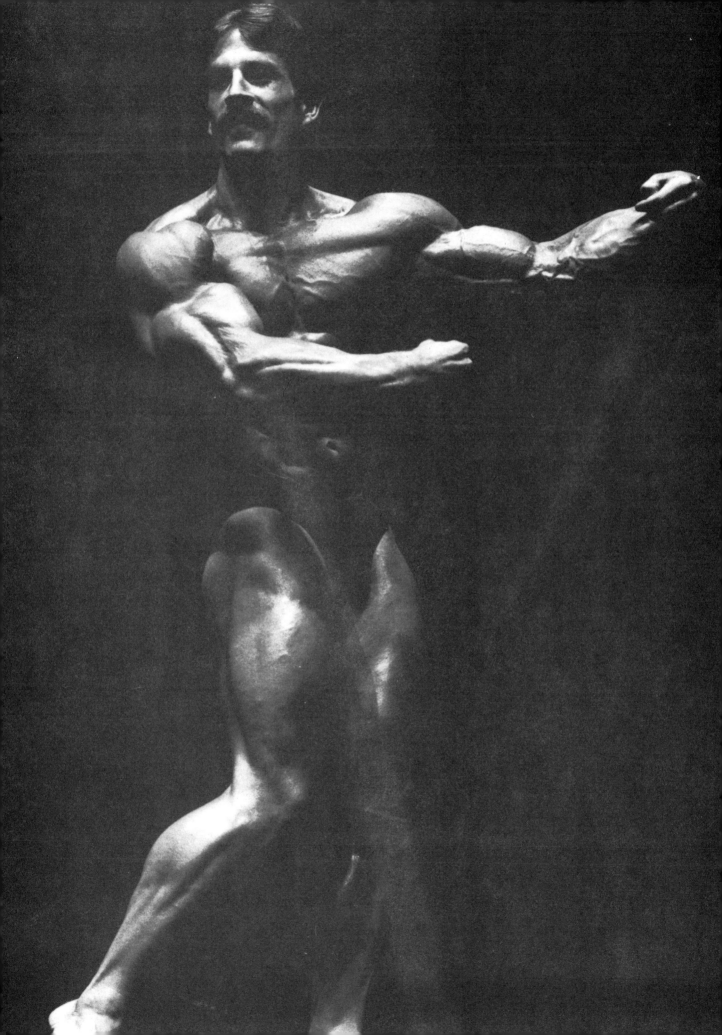

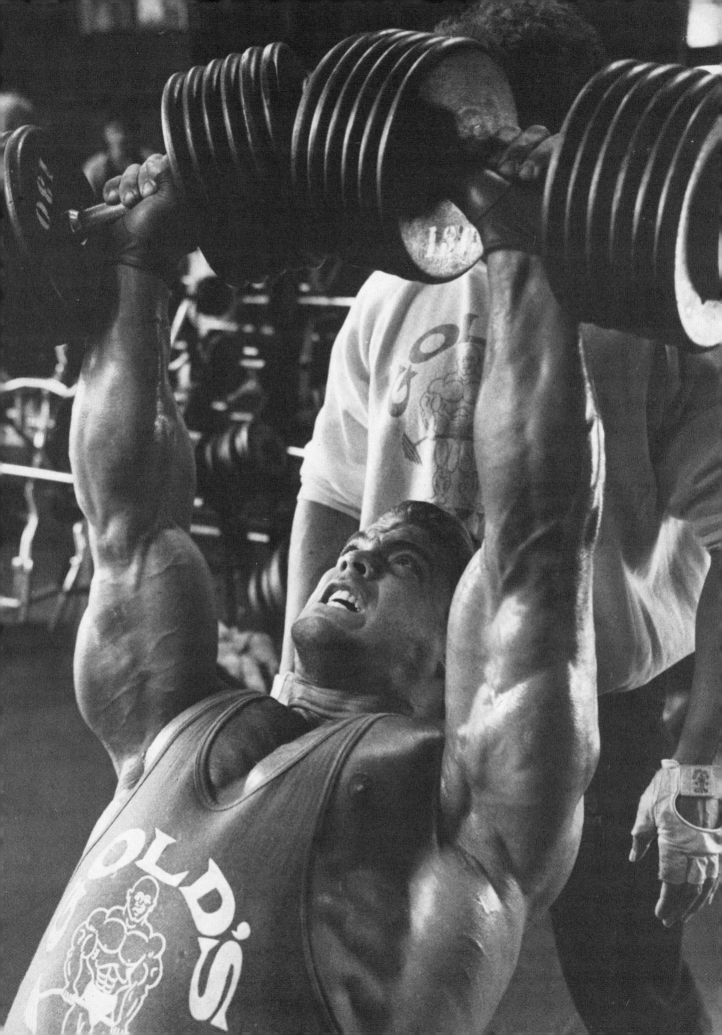

# 6

# How to *Really* Train to Gain

**A**lthough most bodybuilding writers know how to *really* train to stimulate muscle hypertrophy (gain in both muscle mass and strength), few have ever gotten around to writing about how bodybuilding training should be correctly and effectively done. Others write confused garbage about what they think top bodybuilders have told them. You virtually *never* read about how it's *really* done.

Many writers simply haven't trained for competitions or otherwise know very little about bodybuilding, despite indications that they are bright people. Some apparently bright writers choose to push an ineffective system because they can make it seem like it's a very easy way to gain muscle mass. But most of the others write about certain types of routines that will only work for a man whose system is saturated with enough anabolic steroids to embalm a large Irish setter. Little of this has anything to do with how virtually everyone who is making gains naturally (without drugs) is actually going about it.

◄ The concentration needed to build Luiz Freitas into a World Champion was phenomenal. Luiz is another advocate of Zen bodybuilding.

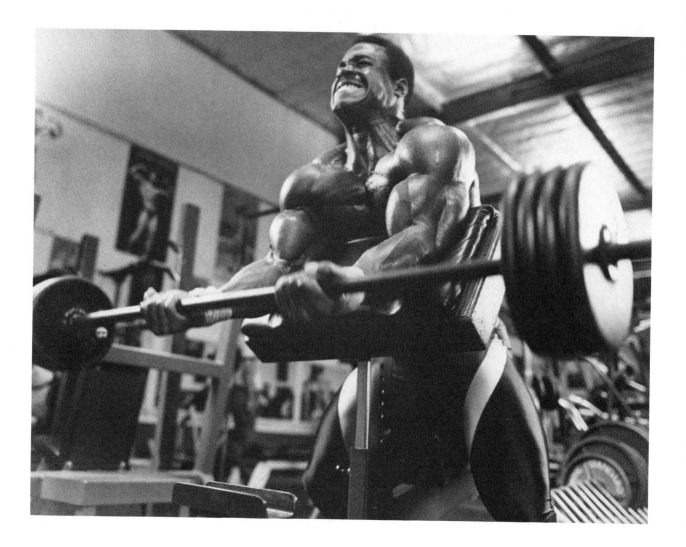

Michael Ashley does some preacher curls.

## The High-Intensity Approach

One author constantly advocates low numbers of sets per body part and very high training intensity during three or four weekly workouts. He says his system is the most scientific. He has fantastic photos of all of the top champs in his books, making a young bodybuilder believe he can look like those big guys on 60 minutes of total training per week. But the real champions don't train this way.

Following are some of the many disadvantages of this brand of high-intensity training:

- It works only for a very small percentage of bodybuilders who can mentally and physically push themselves to the absolute limit on every set.
- Injuries are quite common, since very little warm-up time is allowed and, in an effort to add weight to the bar, body mechanics suffer. I personally know of scores of young bodybuilders who have been seriously injured training this way.

Boyer Coe weighed 217 pounds when this photo was taken two weeks prior to the 1985 Mr. Olympia competition.

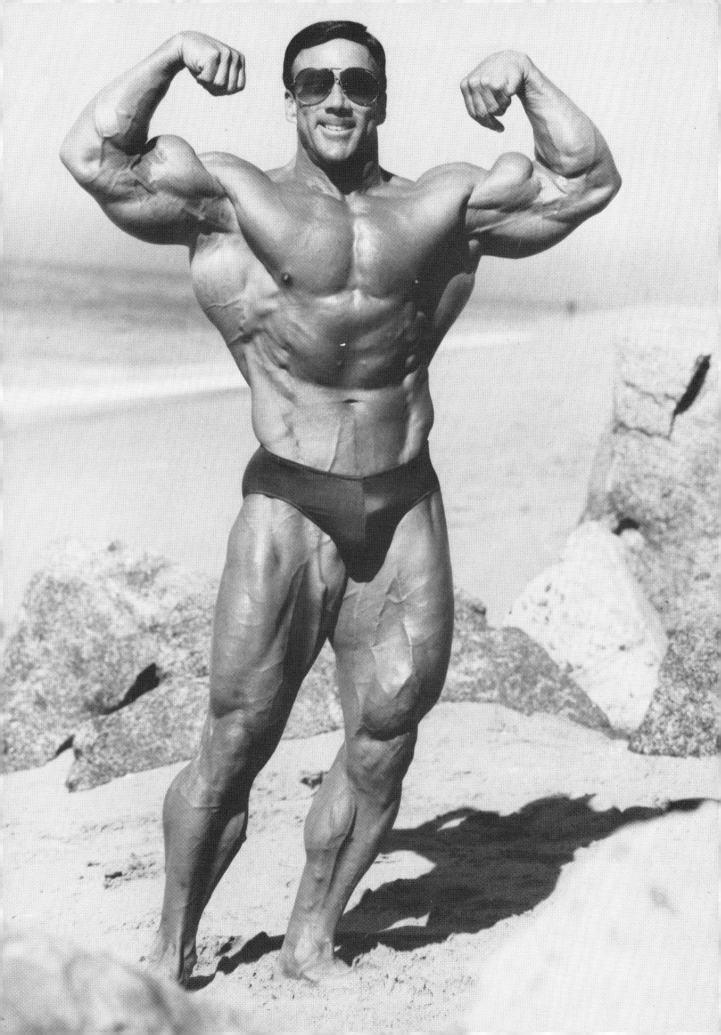

- You will always need a training partner, and you both should work out in a gym that has plenty of Nautilus equipment.
- Those rare few bodybuilders who have built up through high-intensity training usually had great muscle mass and good separation between muscle groups, but very little intramuscular detail.
- One top star who followed the previously mentioned author's suggested high-intensity system to the limit for a year—often with the author supervising his workouts—started the year weighing a hard 210 pounds, but gradually lost muscle mass over the course of his year on the system, ending up weighing barely 180 pounds.

The appeal of this low-sets/high-intensity program is obvious. If a star bodybuilder tells you that you can look just like him, training 2 hours per day six days a week, and a book author writes that you can accomplish the same muscle gains on three or four 20-minute sessions per week, which system would you choose to follow? Why, the easy one, the one in which you'd only have to train 1–1¼ hours per week rather than 12 hours.

The low-sets/high-intensity training might work well for a very few bodybuilders—three former Mr. America winners have been publicized as advocates at various times, while it is well known that they each built up mainly with high-sets workouts—but for most bodybuilders the system is

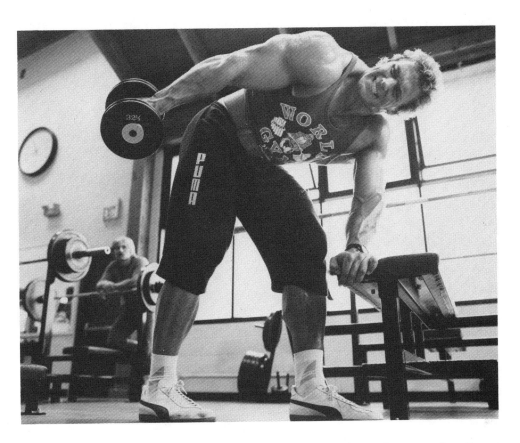

a waste of time and causes numerous joint, muscle and connective tissue injuries.

## The High-Sets Approach

A better training approach—although still not a good one for most natural-training bodybuilders—is the near-daily 2- to 2½-hour workouts featuring twenty to thirty total sets for each muscle group. There's no doubt about it, this is the training system that built *all* of the bodies on view in the high-intensity training books previously mentioned, as well as *all* of the bodies you see in *all* of the bodybuilding magazines.

These men and women used high sets to develop every quality of a bodybuilding champion—great muscle mass, well-balanced physical proportions, sensational body symmetry and the sharpest possible muscle details. But all but a handful of them did not have the incredible natural recovery ability required to recuperate between workouts and actually make progress in building muscle mass.

It is no secret that almost all of the champs in the past twenty years or so who have developed such sensational physiques on high-set workouts were able to do so only by taking varying dosages of androgenic and/or anabolic drugs. Steroids. Long, high-set workouts totally exhaust the body's ability to recover fully between workouts, something I absolutely guarantee is necessary before muscle growth can ever occur.

The *only* way a bodybuilder can foster sufficient recovery ability to grow

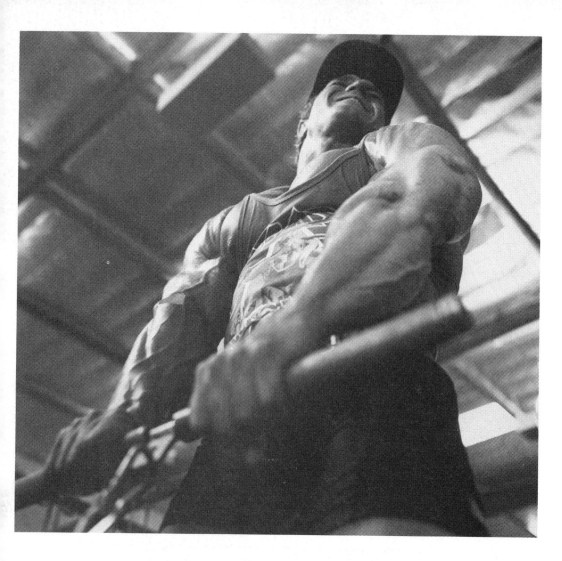

on workouts consisting of twenty to thirty sets per body part—particularly when training six days per week, frequently even twice a day—is to use heavy dosages of anabolic drugs. Anabolics do help to build muscle mass, but this is largely due to their ability to promote fast recovery between long, exhausting workouts.

The reason why high-set workouts are so popular is that they *do* work if you're willing to risk the many side effects attendant to heavy anabolic steroid use. Young bodybuilders think, "Well, if it was good enough to build the physiques of champions A, B and C, it's good enough for me. And getting good enough to win a major title and begin making money off the sport is worth the 'minimal' risk." I've never seen anyone die from taking steroids! is a popular battle cry.

Well, *are* the "minimal" risks okay by you? Are you willing to have your liver and kidneys virtually fall out on the gym floor? Are you willing to watch your testicles shrink to the size of peas, usually making you temporarily sterile in the process? Are you willing to become either sexually impotent or as priapic as a rabbit because of the steroids you're using? Do you want your blood pressure to go off the scale? Do you want so

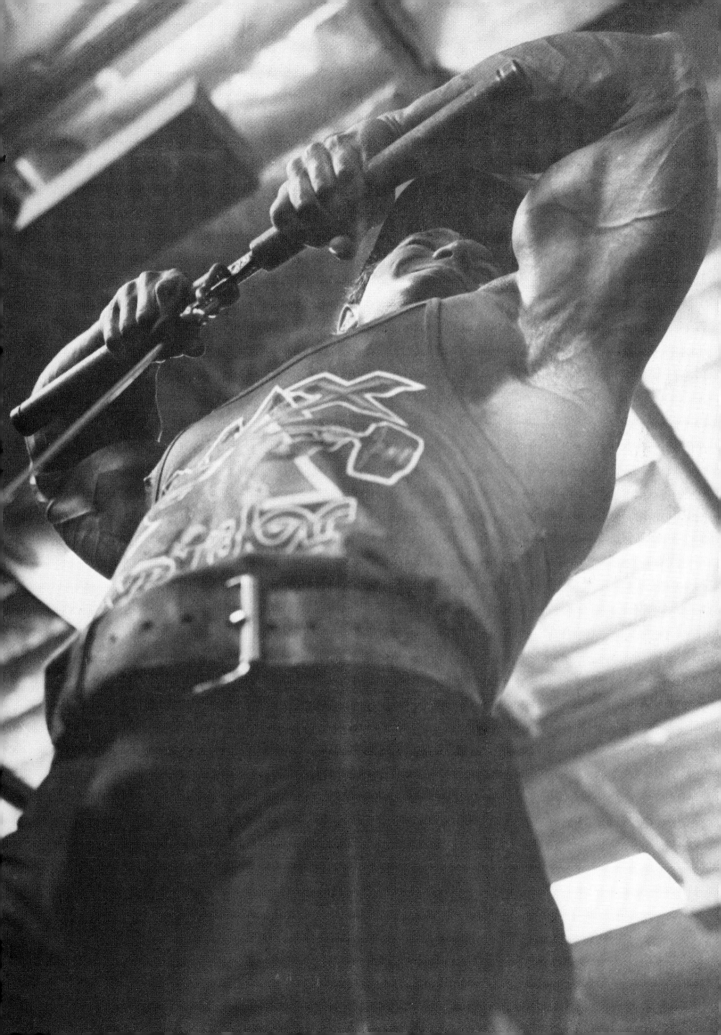

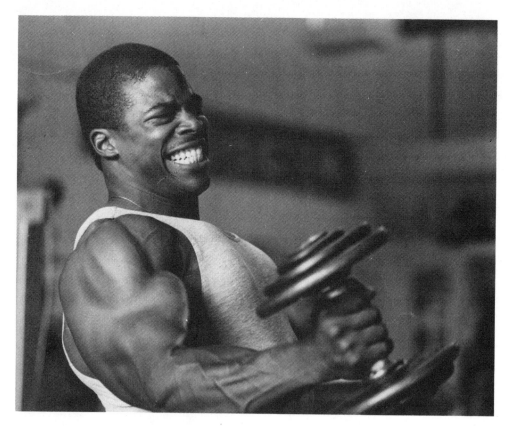

many zits all over your body that you look like you've been machine gunned? And most of all, are you ready to *die* for a few extra pounds of muscle, a half inch more on your biceps?

Bodybuilders *do* die from taking steroids. A shocking number have developed terminal liver tumors because of steroid use. They're now pumping iron in the big gym in the sky. It doesn't have dumbbells higher than 60s, so you might not like it up there.

Bodybuilders also have died of stroke brought on by high blood pressure. And the incredible mood swings—from "I don't give a shit about anything" to "You're dead, man!"—have actually led to well-documented crime sprees, even murder, and to hundreds of undocumented divorces. What 120-pound woman wants to get knocked across the room by a moody 230-pounder who can bench 500 pounds virtually any workout?

The FDA and FBI have been effectively cracking down on illegal steroid sales—those made by pushers in gyms—by arresting "wholesalers" who supply those pushers. The IFBB has been testing women competitors for steroids and other drugs since 1985, men since 1986. The supply of drugs is dropping drastically, and the number of young bodybuilders deciding to train without drugs has skyrocketed to the point where many natural shows are better attended than ones that aren't drug tested.

Natural bodybuilders won't have the recovery ability that the steroid users do, so they need a different, more sane training program, a more Zen-related workout routine. It follows.

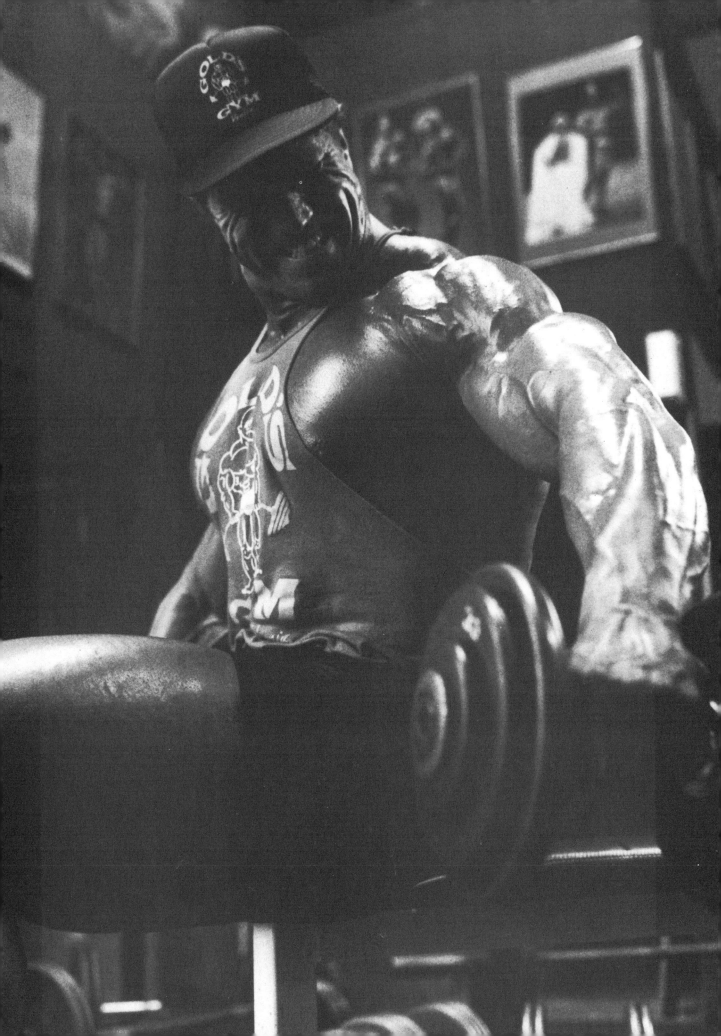

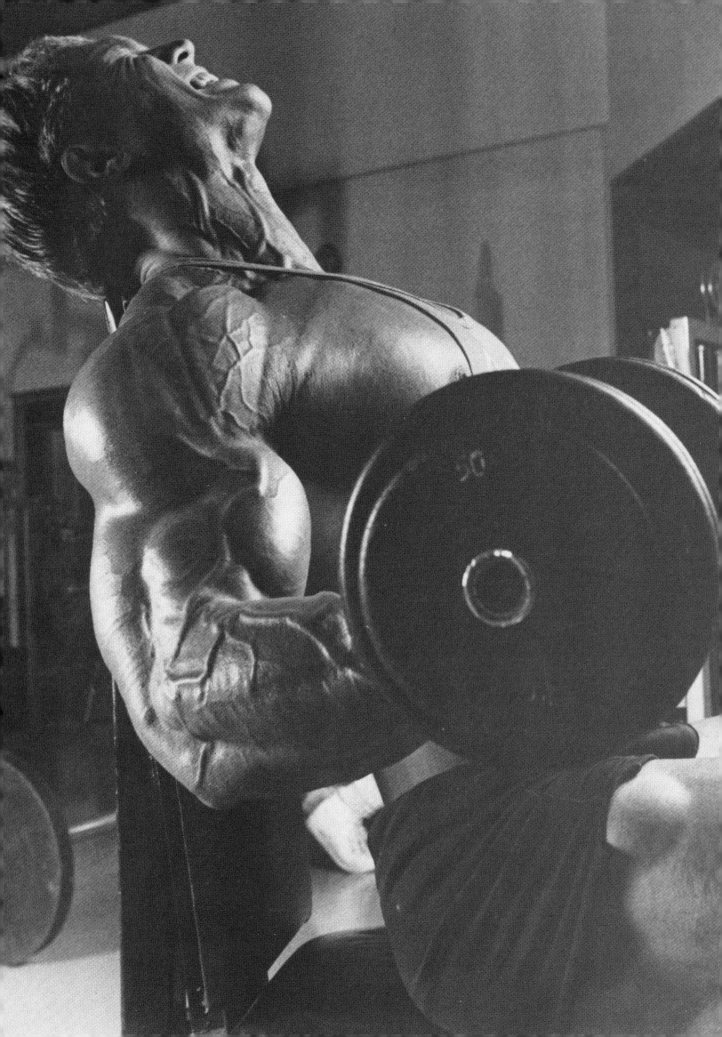

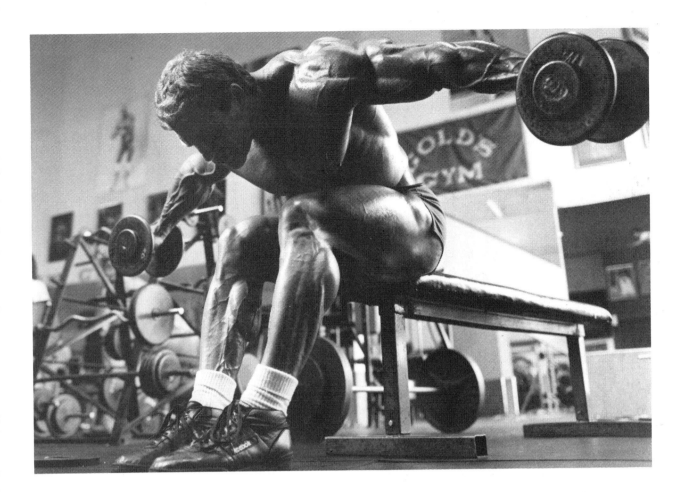

Seated bent-over
laterals with Scott
Wilson.

## The Middle-of-the-Road Zen Approach

Most young bodybuilders are ignorant of the recovery cycle between training sessions, and frequently overtrain as a consequence of their ignorance. It is absolutely axiomatic in the sport that *a muscle cannot and will not increase in mass and strength until after it has completely recovered from its previous workout.* This axiom is so vitally important that you should print it up on a couple of file cards, fastening one to the bathroom mirror and the other to the door of your refrigerator. That way you'll always be aware that lack of recovery time between workouts spells lack of muscle-mass gains.

Since it's so vitally important, let's discuss the recovery cycle. It's very much like your checking account. You deposit money in your checking account each payday and write checks during the weeks between pay periods. Money flows in and money flows out of the account. And as long as you don't write checks for more cash than you have in your account, it remains in balance and the bank is happy with you. The bankers only get on your case when you inadvertently overdraw your checking account. Then they *really* get pissed off at you.

Your body has a dynamic energy expenditure-recovery cycle that works much like your checking account. Energy is deposited in your system as a

Big Gary Strydom
does seated dumb-
bell curls.

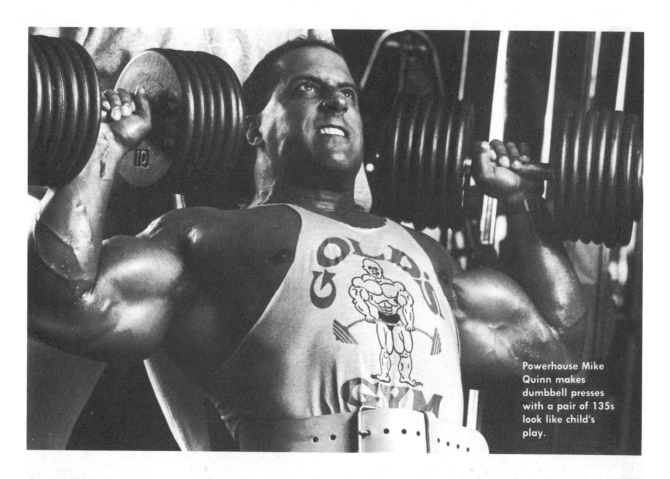

Powerhouse Mike Quinn makes dumbbell presses with a pair of 135s look like child's play.

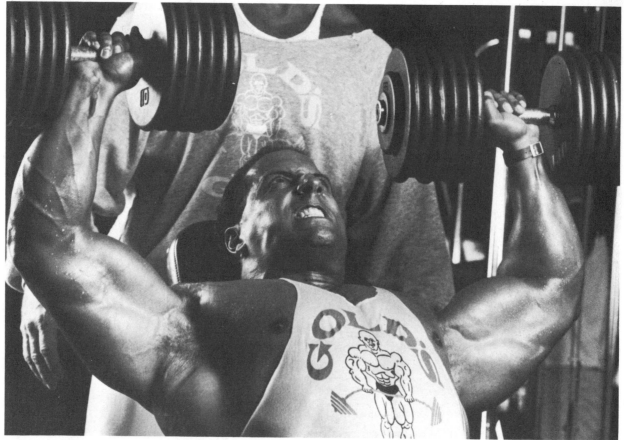

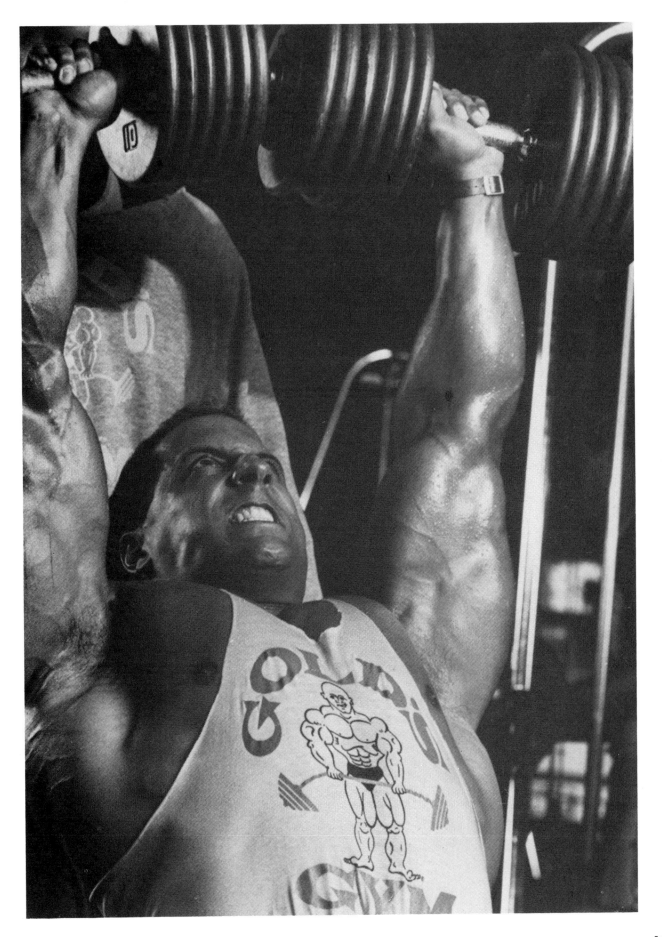

result of following a good diet, getting plenty of sleep and rest, and plugging potential nervous-energy leaks (e.g., depression, feelings of excessive aggression, job anxiety, interpersonal relationships that aren't working out, and so forth).

As with the checking account from which you pay the supermarket, plumber, newspaper boy, you expend energy from that supply as you attempt to build up your workouts even higher each day than the previous one. The primary (and worst) energy drain is excessively long workouts taken almost daily. You can expend too much energy by doing excessive aerobic training as well. And you can expend it by being chronically nervous, failing to sleep and rest enough, and by following a badly balanced, high-junk-food diet.

To digress a bit, I can give you two examples of bodybuilders who did excessive aerobics, and who have admitted it. The first is broad-shouldered Scott Wilson (Pro Mr. International), who was stationary cycling up to 3 hours per day before shows, wondering why he was losing muscle mass, and even muscle density and definition. It also didn't help matters that he was doing forty-five to fifty sets for each major muscle group. Today Scott is back making good gains by doing *no* aerobics and only a fraction as many sets. He was simply burning up so much energy prior to each show that he became chronically run-down and overtrained.

The second individual is Dominique Dardé (IFBB Heavyweight World Champion), who with her husband owns a gym in Rodez, France. After she won the '85 World Championship with a superb physique, everyone in the sport felt she would do well in the pro shows upcoming. But at each one in 1986 her development regressed. She appeared to become progressively smaller and less defined.

Then Dominique made a sensational leap forward with her physique and jumped up to third place at the '87 Pro Worlds, losing out only to Bev Francis (who won) and awesome young Anja Langer. After that championship, I asked Dardé how she had made such stupendous gains. "I finally discovered I was completely wearing myself out teaching four to five 1-hour aerobics classes per day at our gym," she answered. "So we hired a woman to take over the aerobics class load, and I began improving my physique so quickly it was difficult to believe what I was seeing in the mirror!"

The message here is that you can overtrain by doing too much aerobic training, as well as by spending too many hours in the gym pumping iron. But the main culprit by far in the overtraining equation is always excessively long bodybuilding sessions.

Training too frequently is also a common cause of becoming overtrained. A six-day split routine is de rigueur with virtually all top bodybuilders. A handful of men and women actually double-split their routines, taking two workouts per day, one in the morning and the other late in the afternoon or early in the evening. But if you're not taking drugs, and lots of them, your chances are zero that you'll avoid overtraining and make gains on a six-day split.

### Split Routines

How many workouts should you take per week? If you are a beginner (a person with less than six months of steady, progressively more intense gym sessions), you should train your entire physique in one session on three nonconsecutive days per week. All other natural bodybuilders should either follow a four-day split routine or a program in which they train three straight days and then take two days to rest before beginning the five-day cycle anew.

The four-day split routine is a bit less intense than the three-on/two-off program. Here is a sample four-day split routine:

| *Monday-Thursday* | *Tuesday-Friday* |
|---|---|
| Abdominals | Calves |
| Chest | Legs |
| Back | Upper Arms |
| Shoulders | Forearms |

You have probably noticed that I haven't mentioned doing any neck training in this routine. Virtually all young bodybuilders achieve excellent neck development simply as a consequence of the exercises they perform for muscle groups adjacent to the neck—upper chest, upper back and shoulders.

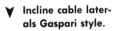
▼ Incline cable laterals Gaspari style.

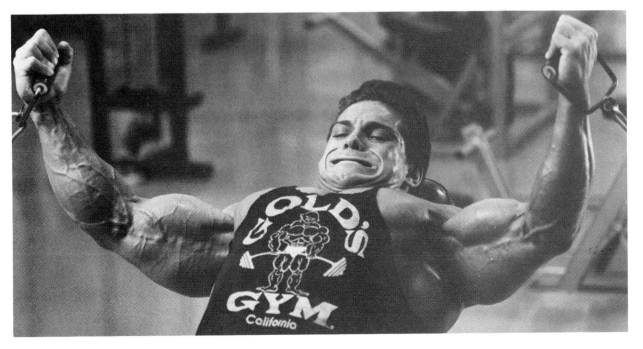

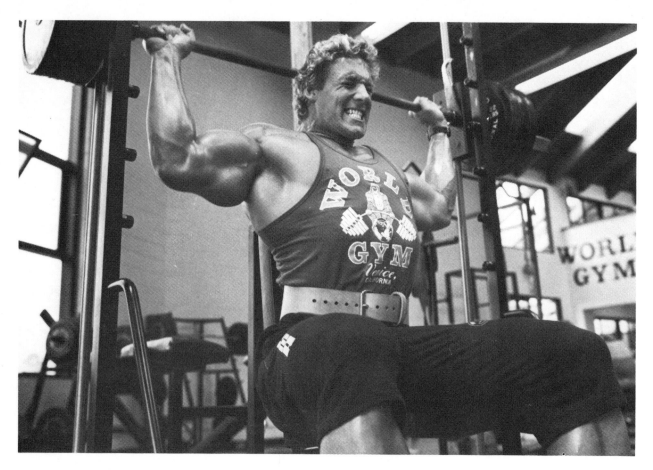

When you follow a four-day split system, your workout days occur only during the week, leaving weekends free. With the five-day cycle, however, you will frequently have to train on weekends. But this shouldn't deter any serious bodybuilder from using the five-day cycle program.

Following is one example of how you can split up your body parts for the five-day split-routine cycle:

| Day 1 | Day 2 | Day 3 | Day 4 | Day 5 |
|-------|-------|-------|-------|-------|
| Abdominals | Quads | Calves | Rest | Rest |
| Chest | Hamstrings | Middle Back | | |
| Shoulders | Lower Back | Upper Back | | |
| Triceps | Forearms | Biceps | | |

Both of the foregoing split routines will work wonders for your physique as long as exercises are correctly chosen and you adhere to the parameters I will give you for total sets on each muscle group. Oh, yes. You also must use Zen to tap your strongest inner resources to help you keep constantly increasing the weight you can use with strict form in each movement.

## Basic Exercises

The backbone of any natural mass-building routine must be the use of basic exercises rather than isolation exercises. For the sake of definition, an *isolation exercise* is one which places stress on a single specific muscle

Luiz Freitas doing ➤
incline dumbbell
presses.

group—sometimes even on just part of that complex—without the help of other muscles, which are often stronger than the group being isolated. Isolation movements are best used during a contest peaking cycle, when your objective is to maintain existing muscle mass while shaping and defining individual body parts.

In direct contrast, a *basic exercise* works the larger muscle complexes in your body (legs, back, chest) with help from other muscle groups. Basic movements, as I hinted, are best used in heavy training to increase muscle mass.

Let me give you one isolation movement and one basic exercise for the same muscle group, so you can compare them. Doing flyes on a pec deck machine isolates the stress primarily on the pectorals with only slight help from the anterior delts. And over the second half of the movement, pec deck flyes place much greater stress on the inner pecs than those parts of the muscle out toward the shoulder joints.

You could also work your pectorals with heavy bench presses, one of the best basic exercises for the chest and the rest of the upper body. Benches do work pectorals quite intensely, and the front delts and triceps intensely as well. Benches even stress the lats and those upper back muscles that impart rotational force to the scapulae when the arms are extended upward. As such, the bench press is an excellent basic exercise.

For your convenience, you will find a list of the best basic exercises for each body part in Figure 1 on page 126.

The object when mass building—whether you are natural or take a metric ton of steroids—is to use primarily basic exercises in your routines,

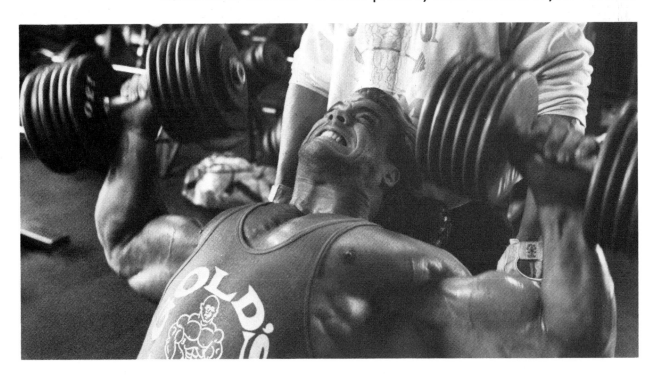

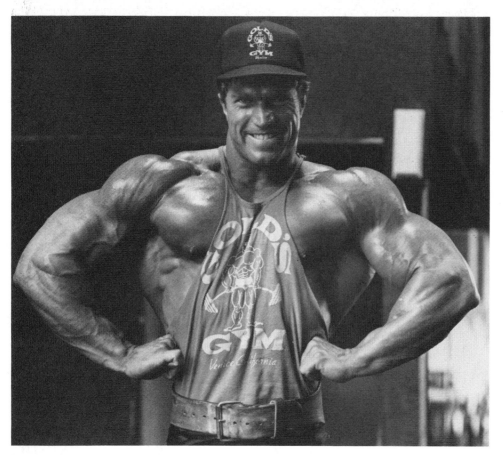

▲ Gary Strydom.

### Figure 1: The Best Basic Exercises

| Muscle Group | Basic Exercises |
|---|---|
| Quadriceps | Squats, Front Squats, Leg Presses at various angles |
| Hamstrings | Stiff-Legged Deadlifts |
| Lower Back | Deadlifts |
| Middle Back | Chins, Pulldowns, Cable Rows, Barbell and Dumbbell Rows |
| Upper Back | Shrugs, Upright Rows |
| Pectorals | Bench Presses, Incline Presses, Decline Presses, Parallel Bar Dips |
| Deltoids | All forms of overhead pressing (machine, barbell, dumbbells), Upright Rows |
| Biceps | Standing Barbell Curls, Barbell Preacher Curls, Standing or Seated Dumbbell Curls |
| Triceps | Parallel Bar Dips (torso held erect), Close-Grip Bench Presses, all forms of overhead pressing |
| Forearms | Barbell Reverse Curls, Standing Barbell Wrist Curls |
| Abdominals | Hanging Leg Raises, Sit-Ups |
| Calves | Standing Calf Raises, Seated Calf Raises |

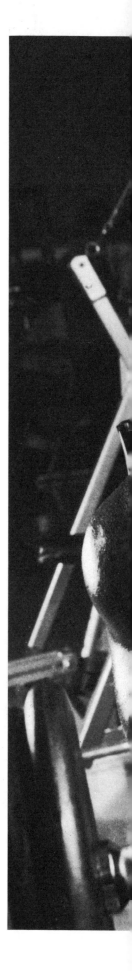

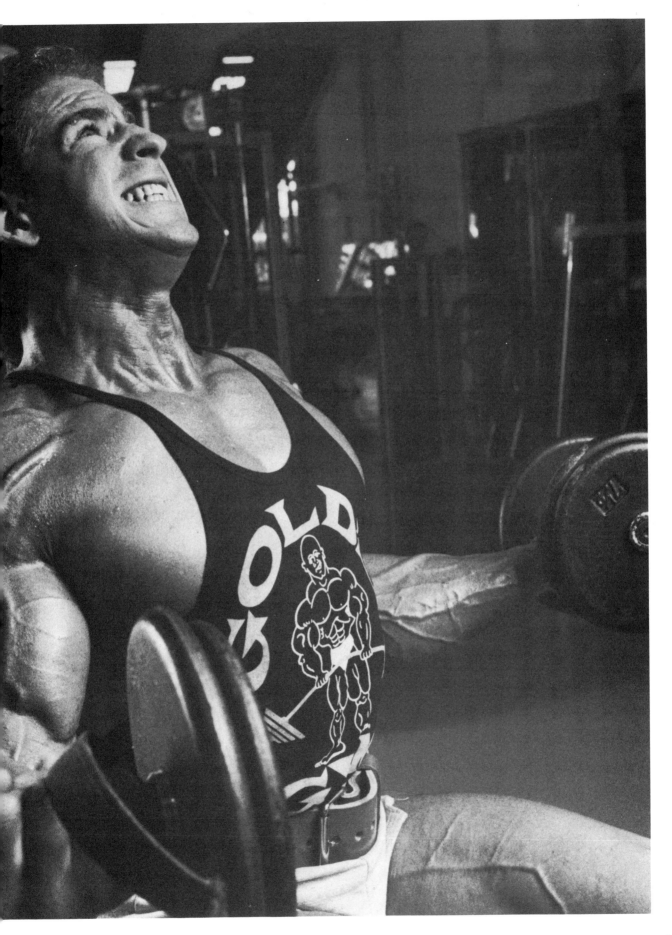

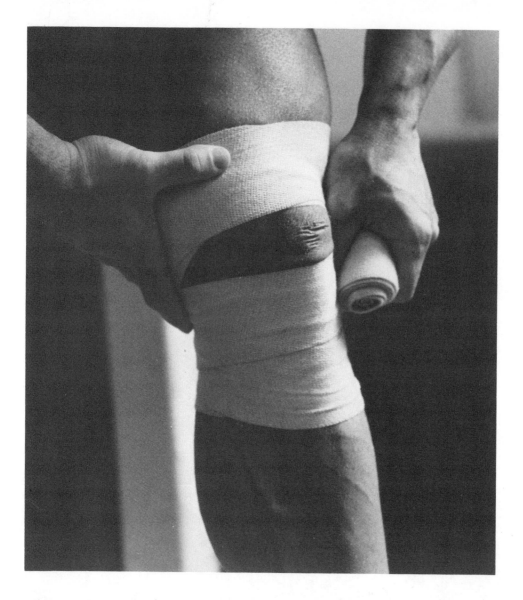

using maximum weights in each set with optimum biomechanics (body form). And once you've started competing, you'll always return to basic exercises during the off-season to add general muscle mass to your physique.

Here are two closing comments from superstar bodybuilders about basic exercises that should interest you:

- Boyer Coe (IFBB Pro World Grand Prix Champion) says, "I never did anything for my legs except squats three times per week until I had won the Mr. America title."

- Dennis Tinerino (IFBB Pro Mr. Universe) reveals, "Every young bodybuilder should train entirely on basic exercises for at least three years. That's the only way you can get your basic muscle mass up to the level where using isolation work would be of any value. You can't shape muscle mass that you don't already have."

## Pyramid Power

"In order to build large, powerful muscles," reveals Mike Christian (World Pro Champion, 1988), "you must concentrate on lifting very heavy weights for relatively low reps, all in perfect form. But you also need to warm up your joints and muscles with lighter poundages and higher reps in order to avoid injuries with the really heavy weights.

"The best solution I know of that meets these mass-building criteria is to pyramid—or half-pyramid—your weights and reps. With each succeeding set you increase the weight by 10–15 pounds—up to 30–50 pounds for some leg and back movements—while correspondingly decreasing reps. You eventually get up to a maximum weight for four or five very intense repetitions. Then you can leave it at that, or do one down set for an extra high-rep pump. This involves dropping the poundage about 40–50 percent from your highest effort, then pumping out as many reps as possible with the lighter poundage."

▼ The massive German Ralf Moeller hits alternate dumbbell curls at the new World Gym.

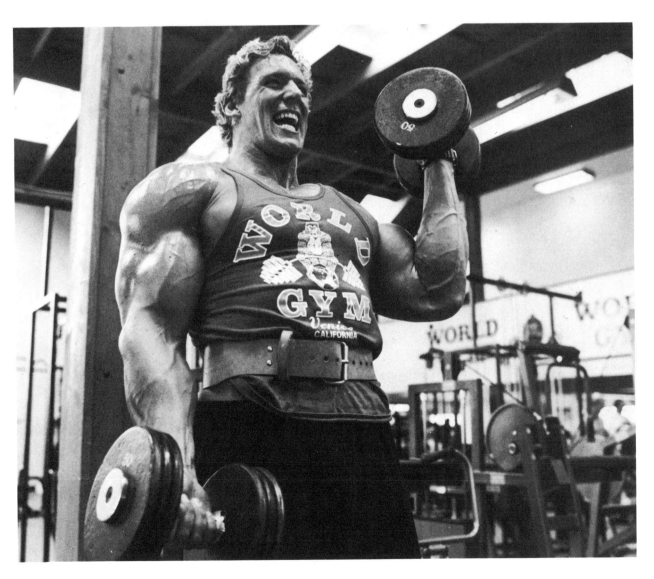

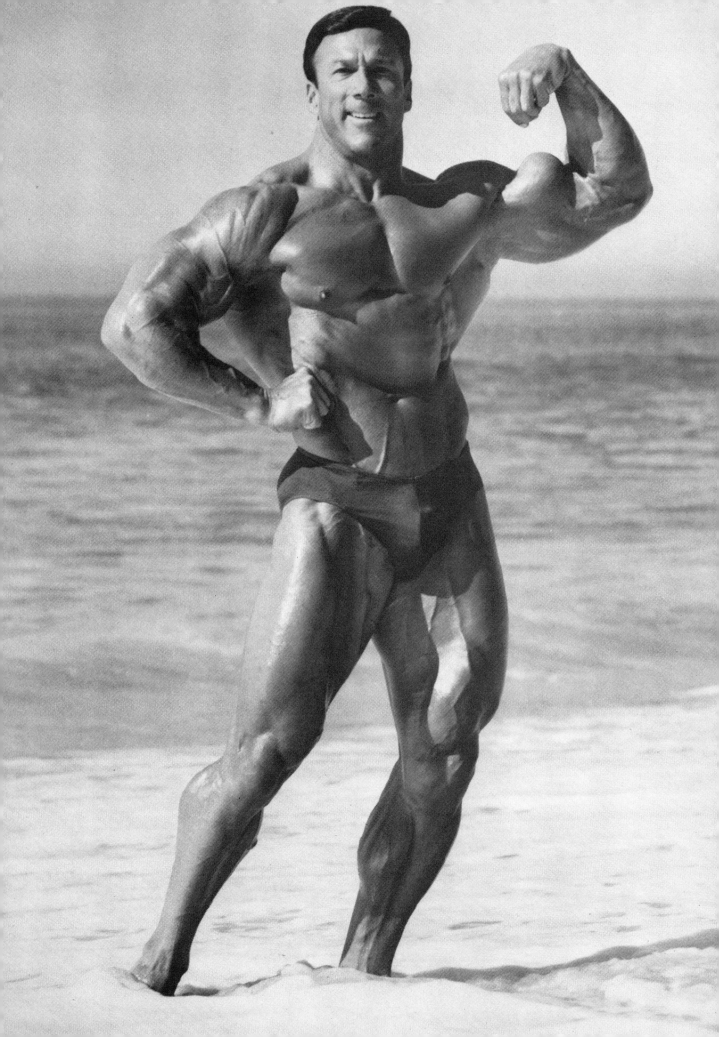

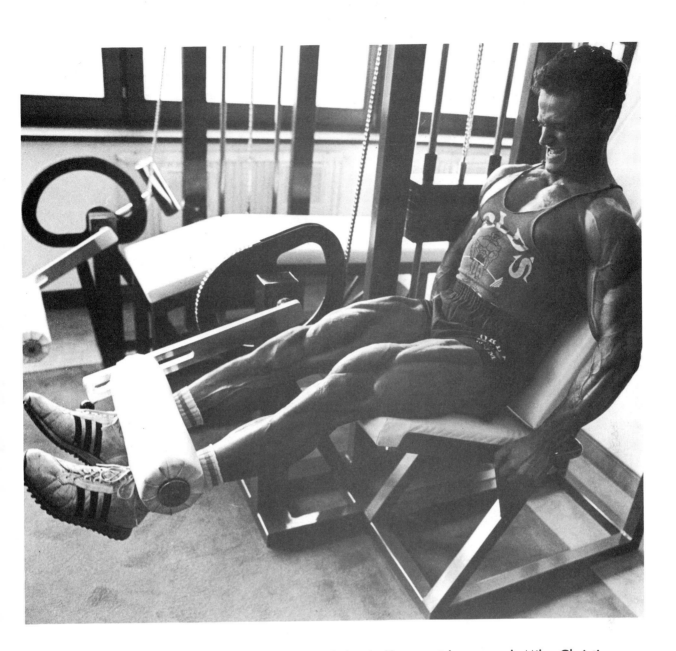

▲ Leg extensions are needed to build the muscles above the knee.

Following is a table of this half-pyramid approach Mike Christian recommends, using barbell incline presses for the movement (weights are arbitrarily selected solely for the purpose of illustration):

| Set Number | Weight (lbs.) | Number of Reps |
|---|---|---|
| 1 | 135 | 12 |
| 2 | 165 | 10 |
| 3 | 190 | 8 |
| 4 | 205 | 6 |
| 5 | 220 | 4–5 |
| 6 | 155 | 12–15 |

This pyramid power method works quite well as long as you keep pushing the weights on all of your basic exercises while maintaining perfect biomechanics (form). I wouldn't recommend pyramiding abdominal exercises, however; straight sets will do just fine for that body part.

◄ Boyer Coe at Muscle Beach.

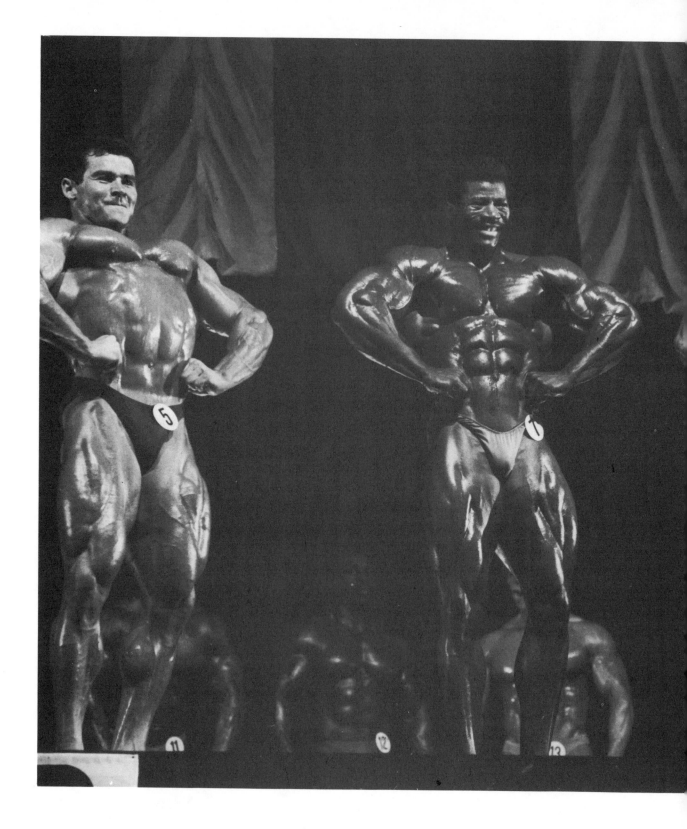

## My Recommended Routines

Long and occasional painful experience has convinced me that most advanced bodybuilders training naturally can make optimum progress doing no more than ten to twelve total sets for large muscle groups and no more than six to eight total sets for smaller body parts. You can treat the back

Left to right: Josef Grolmus, Ron Love and Ed Kawak at the 1987 IFBB Pro World Championships.

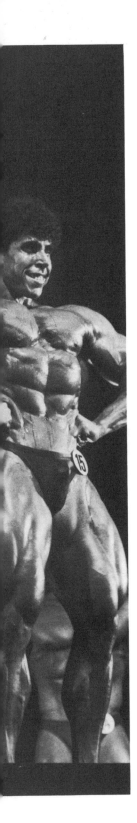

as either two or three muscle groups, however, since it is such a large and complex area of your body. Quads and hamstrings each are one large muscle group, a total of two muscle complexes to be trained heavy and hard; biceps and triceps count as one small body part each.

Everything but abdominals will be pyramided, and it's essential that you have an alert training partner standing by as a safety spotter on maximum-weight sets, particularly of bench presses and squats. On the highest two or three sets of each pyramided exercise, you should go to failure, with perhaps one solid forced rep here and there. But don't overdo the forced reps. Most bodybuilders overtrain when they push too many sets *past* the failure point, using forced reps or any other method.

Following are two suggested routines, one four-day split and one three-on/two-off split. Obviously you can feel free to adapt them to suit your equipment availability. I'd recommend following one for six to eight weeks, or until you grow bored with it, then switch off to the other one, alternating the two for as long a period as you continue to make good gains in muscle mass on them both. *Never* do more than the suggested number of sets in any of the suggested exercises.

### ROUTINE A

#### Monday-Thursday

| Exercise | Sets | Reps |
|---|---|---|
| 1. Hanging Leg Raises | 2–3 | 15–20 |
| 2. Bench Presses | 6 | 12–5* |
| 3. Barbell Incline Presses | 6 | 12–5* |
| 4. Standing Barbell Presses | 6 | 12–5* |
| 5. Barbell Upright Rows | 6 | 12–5* |
| 6. Lying Barbell Triceps Extensions | 6 | 12–5* |
| 7. Standing Barbell Curls | 6 | 12–5* |
| 8. Seated Calf Raises | 6 | 15–8* |

#### Tuesday-Friday

| Exercise | Sets | Reps |
|---|---|---|
| 1. Incline Sit-Ups | 2–3 | 20–30 |
| 2. Squats | 6 | 12–5* |
| 3. Angled Leg Presses | 5 | 12–5* |
| 4. Stiff-Legged Deadlifts | 6 | 15–8* |
| 5. Back Hyperextensions (weighted) | 4 | 10–15 |
| 6. Seated Pulley Rows | 6 | 12–5* |
| 7. Front Lat Machine Pulldowns | 6 | 12–5* |
| 8. Standing Barbell Reverse Curls | 5 | 12–6* |
| 9. Standing Calf Raises | 6 | 20–10* |

*Note:* Pyramid all exercises marked with an asterisk, including the down (pump) sets whenever doing six sets of a movement.

### Day 1

| Exercise | Sets | Reps |
|---|---|---|
| 1. Roman Chair Sit-Ups | 2–3 | 50 |
| 2. Barbell Incline Presses | 6 | 12–5* |
| 3. Parallel Bar Dips (weighted) | 6 | 15–8* |
| 4. Front Chins (weighted) | 6 | 12–6* |
| 5. Barbell Bent Rows | 6 | 15–8* |
| 6. Barbell Shrugs | 6 | 15–8* |
| 7. Standing Calf Raises | 6 | 15–8* |

### Day 2

| Exercise | Sets | Reps |
|---|---|---|
| 1. Back Hyperextensions (weighted) | 2–3 | 10–15 |
| 2. Squats | 6 | 12–5* |
| 3. Angled Leg Presses | 6 | 15–5* |
| 4. Lying Leg Curls | 5 | 12–6* |
| 5. Stiff-Legged Deadlifts | 4 | 15–8* |
| 6. Standing Barbell Reverse Curls | 5 | 12–6* |

### Day 3

| Exercise | Sets | Reps |
|---|---|---|
| 1. Hanging Leg Raises | 2–3 | 15–20 |
| 2. Seated Presses Behind Neck | 6 | 15–5* |
| 3. Barbell or Cable Upright Rows | 6 | 12–5* |
| 4. Barbell Triceps Extensions | 6 | 12–6* |
| 5. Barbell Preacher Curls | 6 | 12–5* |
| 6. Barbell Wrist Curls | 4 | 10–12 |
| 7. Seated Calf Raises | 6 | 12–6* |

*Note:* Pyramid all exercises marked with an asterisk, including the recommended down (pump) sets whenever doing six sets of a movement.

One-arm rows as done by Gary Strydom.

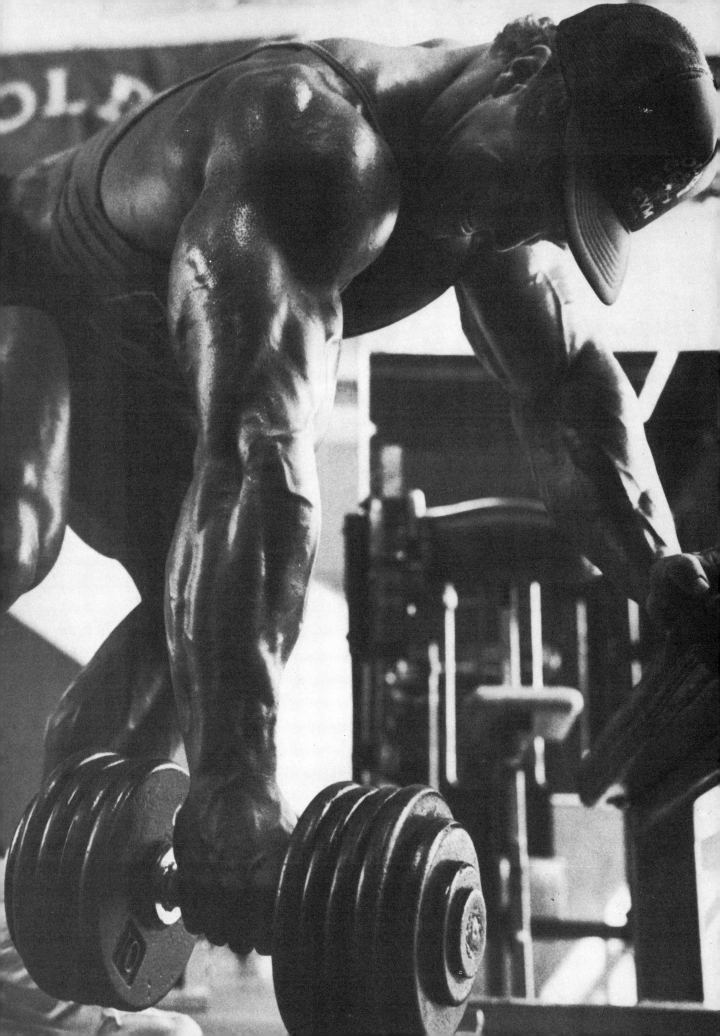

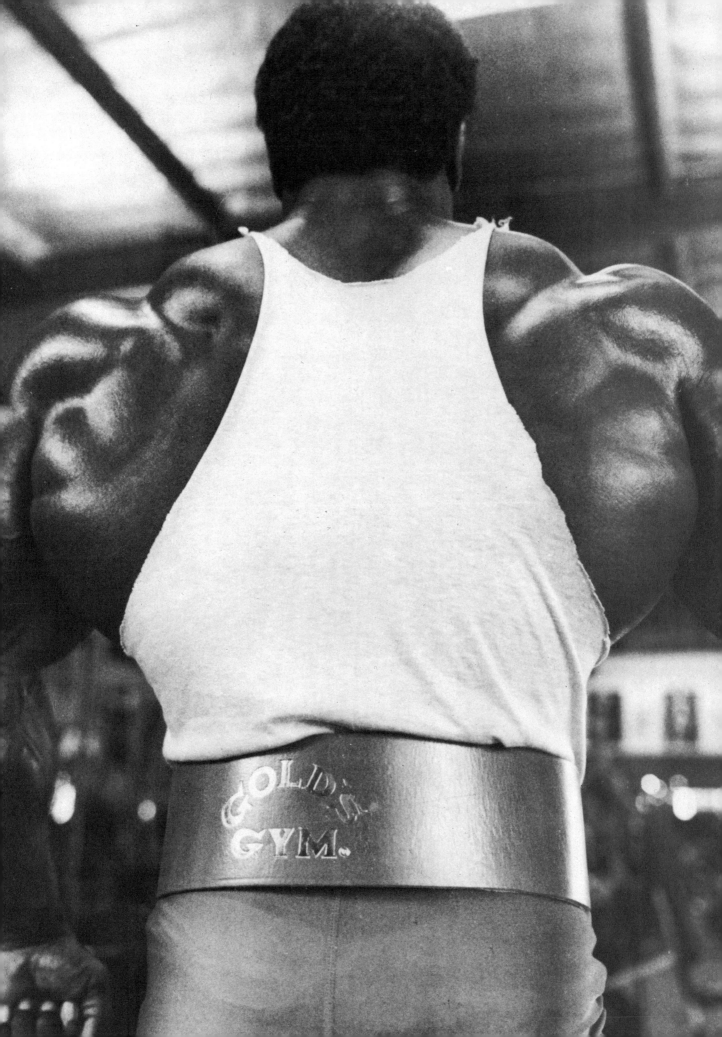

# 7

# Advanced Bodybuilding

**B**eginning and intermediate bodybuilders are concerned almost exclusively with building general muscle mass. Advanced bodybuilders are still preoccupied with increasing general muscle mass, but they must also concentrate their efforts on sharpening other physical qualities which contest judges evaluate onstage. There are six general physical and performance qualities that influence how a judge scores you at each competition, so let's talk about each one in some detail.

- *Proportional Balance.* In competitive bodybuilding—particularly at the pro and high amateur levels of the sport—an even balance of relative muscle mass from one body part to the next is a highly prized quality. All of the most venerated bodybuilding champions have developed physiques with no over- or underdeveloped muscle groups. Invariably, the men with underdeveloped delts or calves and overdeveloped pecs or biceps fail to make it very high in the sport. A few bodybuilders with marginally weak areas are currently competing professionally, but the only men who win major titles are those with nearly perfect proportional balance.

◀ **The most amazing back in bodybuilding: Lee Haney.**

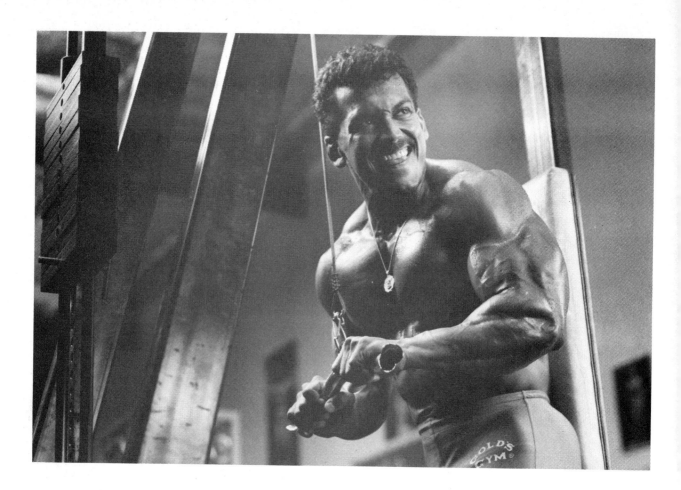

In a few pages I will thoroughly discuss the relatively new cycle training technique in which top-level bodybuilders follow distinct off-season and precontest phases aimed at improving every facet of their physiques. When in an off-season cycle, your two goals should be to increase general muscle mass and to particularly improve the mass and development of a weak muscle group. And during a peaking cycle, your dietary and training efforts should have only one objective—to maintain a maximum degree of muscle mass while dieting off all extraneous body fat.

Toward the end of this chapter, I will present Lee Haney's thoughts on priority training in order to improve a lagging muscle group during an off-season cycle. This discussion will include several tips on how to increase training intensity when specializing on a weak muscle group.

• *Muscle Mass.* Muscle mass is also a vitally important ingredient of a great physique. Casual examination of several contest reports in *Flex* magazine will show you that gradual upward increments in muscle mass are necessary to climb up the ladder of competitive success. At the professional level, all bodybuilders have a great deal of muscle mass, with the current Mr. Olympia, Lee Haney, being the Big Daddy of them all.

Upright row with ➤
Ralf Moeller.

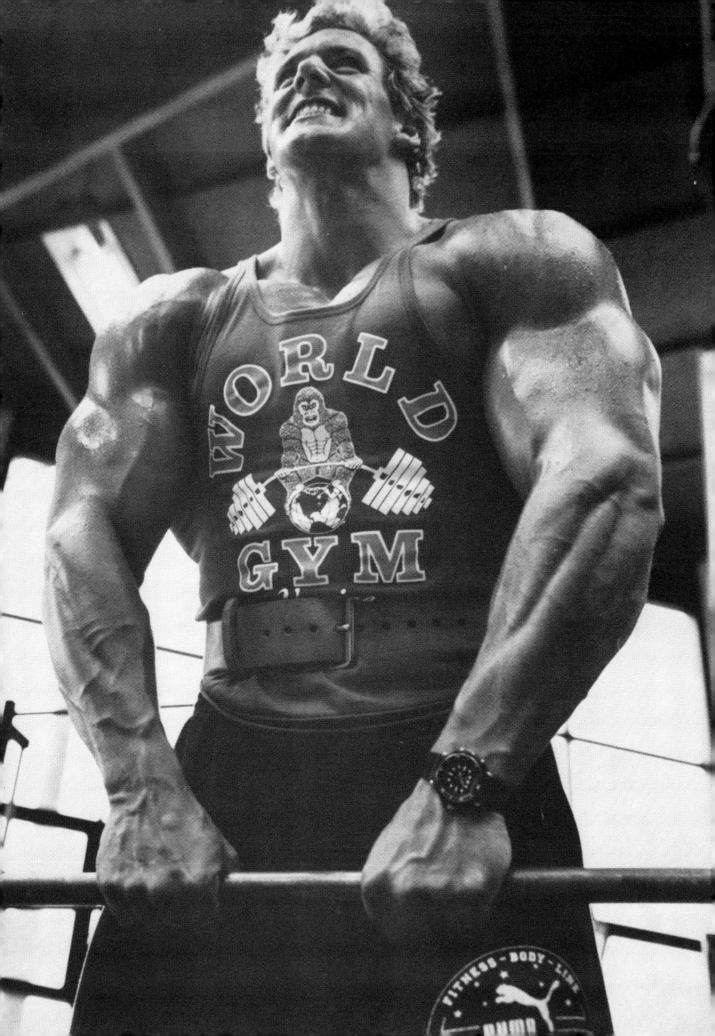

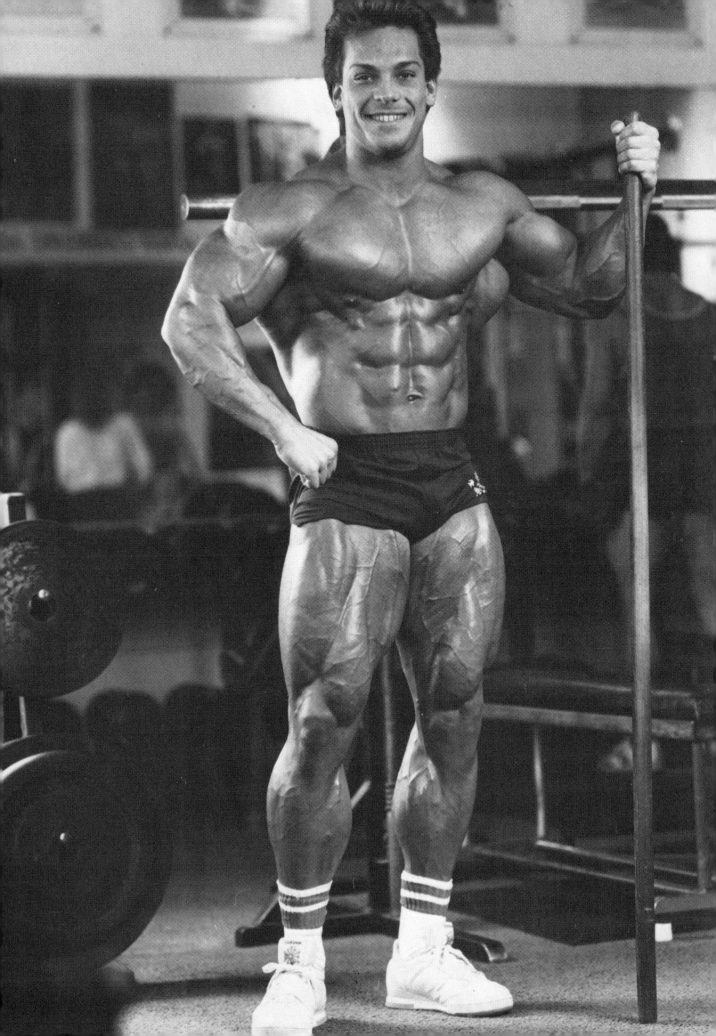

Muscle mass will gradually increase as a consequence of accumulated heavy training. The longer you are in the sport and the longer you have been training consistently hard and heavy, the larger your muscles will become. Obviously, there is an upper limit to how large your muscles can become, although watching Haney year after year has convinced me that no one has yet visualized this upper level for muscle mass. And even Lee has had to be patient as he gradually increased the relative mass of each muscle group.

- *Muscularity.* At contest time an intense degree of muscularity (absence of body fat which obscures muscular development) is essential if you expect to take home any trophy, let alone the biggest one. Look at a few contest reports again, and you'll see that the top guys in all high-level shows are very muscular. There are cuts in their quads so deep that you could almost hide quarters in them!

Any bodybuilder who is willing to pay the price in his diet and level of aerobic training can achieve a high degree of muscular definition. For some it's much more difficult than for others, but everyone can rip up like a champ. Precontest diet is too involved a topic to discuss within the scope of this book, so for further information on this spe-

◄ The superb physique of Rich Gaspari.

▼ Lee Haney doing bent-over dumbbell laterals.

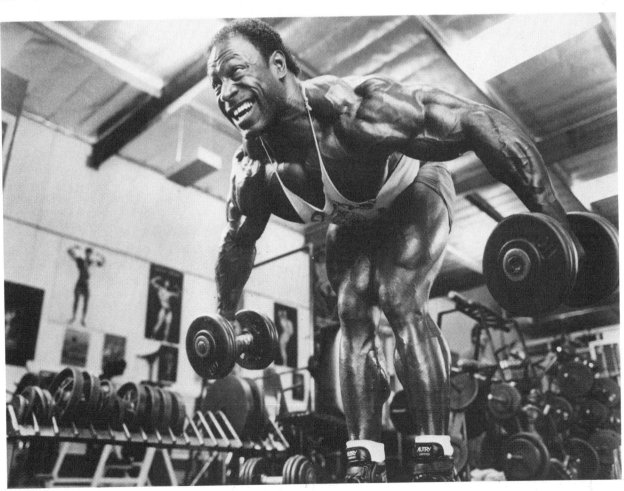

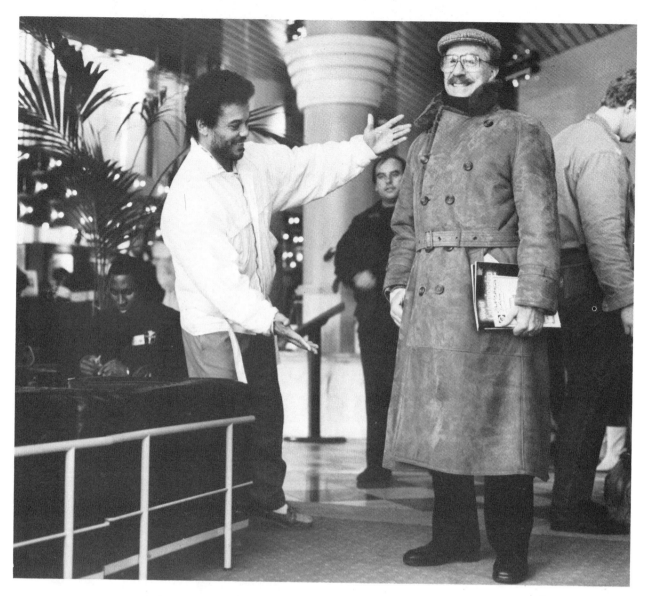

cialized type of nutritional approach, I suggest you read my *Gold's Gym Nutrition Bible.*

- *Symmetry.* When someone writes or talks about a bodybuilder's symmetry, he means the outline of that man's physique, as though seen in silhouette. To possess ideal body symmetry, you should have broad shoulders, flaring lats that taper down to a minuscule waist and hip structure. Ideally you should have relatively small joints (knees, ankles, wrists, etc.) with bulging muscles adjacent to them. Lee Haney has the most ideal symmetry among the current crop of professional competitors.

- *Stage Presence.* The four foregoing qualities are all physical, while stage presence refers to your performance ability onstage, and your general comportment while onstage at both the prejudging and evening show. And you can only develop this type of stage presence through hours of practice. The athletes who are best at it—men such as Shawn

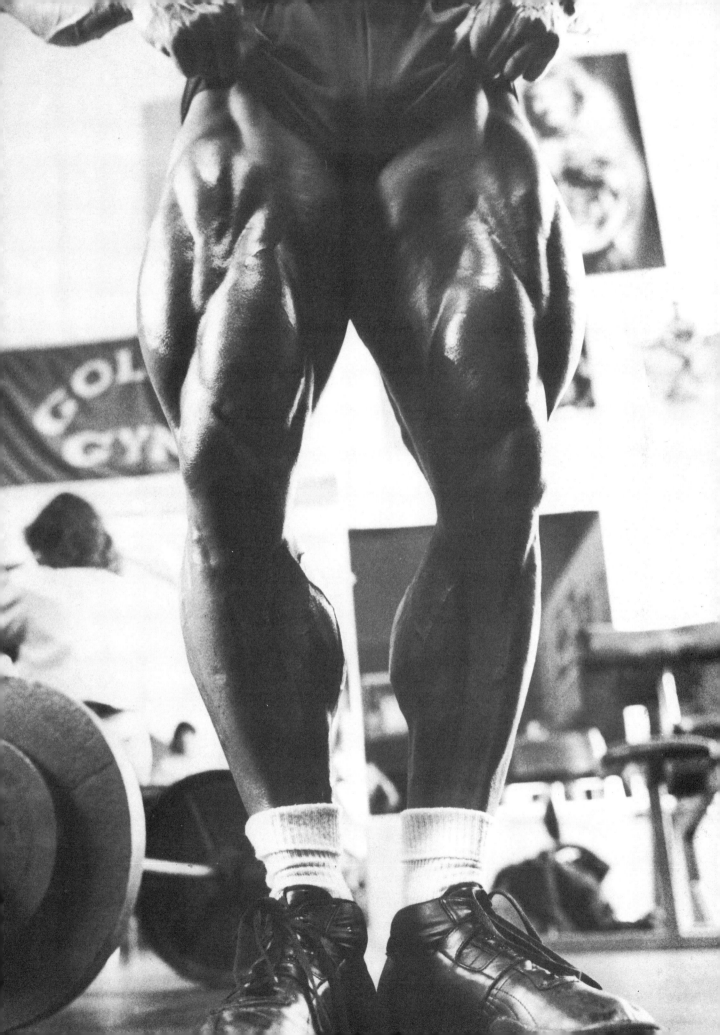

Ray, who won the overall 1987 National Championship at only 22 years of age—practice daily for up to an hour each time, even up to 3–4 hours per day prior to a competition.

- *General Appearance.* This final quality of a championship physique involves perfect personal grooming, attention to tan and skin tone, and choice of posing attire cut and color. It obviously takes far less time to optimize your physical appearance than to develop a contest-winning physique, but this doesn't mean you can leave it until the final week of contest prep. You should begin work on your tan (if you don't come with one built in) and prepare your posing attire at least two to three months before your show.

## Cycle Training

By alternating off-season building cycles with precontest defining cycles, you will ultimately combine both Herculean muscle mass and diamond-hard cuts. A rare bodybuilder from time to time is able to develop both qualities by training and eating the same way year-round, but most top bodybuilders cycle their training and nutritional programs.

The length of off-season and precontest cycles is crucial. Many of the best bodybuilders—Haney, Albert Beckles, Corey Everson and other pros—compete only once a year. This allows them to train heavy and build up muscle mass during a long off-season cycle lasting nine to ten months. Then over the final two to three months they are in their precontest cycle in order to peak for a Mr. or Ms. Olympia show.

Lee Haney says, "One of the reasons I have been able to compete with significantly more muscle mass each succeeding Olympia is the length of my off-season building cycles. I've seen numerous rising young bodybuilders stymie their progress by becoming trophy hungry and entering every competition in sight. I know one potentially great bodybuilder in Atlanta, where I live, who entered fourteen shows in a six-month period of time. He harvested twenty-odd trophies, but was actually losing muscle mass toward the end of his self-imposed ordeal.

"It's impossible to build any real muscle when you're in a peaking mode. At best you can maintain muscle mass while stripping away body fat. So it's essential that you allow yourself sufficient time to build muscle mass between your peaking phases. You'll only be able to train with maximum weights and intensity when you're able to eat enough calories to fuel all-out training sessions, and that only occurs during an off-season cycle.

"When I'm coaching upcoming competitive bodybuilders, I always recommend competing no more frequently than twice a year, preferably with equal, six-month intervals between peaks. This permits building phases lasting 3½–4 months followed by peaking phases lasting 2–2½ months.

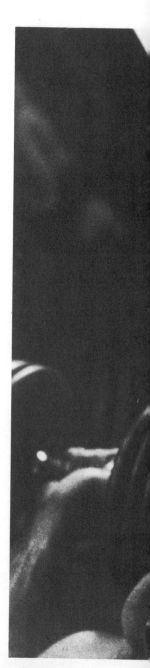

Seated dumbbell press with Gary Strydom.

In this way, you allow yourself sufficient heavy training time between shows to progressively build up your physique and improve weak points.

"If it is possible, peak only once per year, so you can maintain your off-season cycle for nine to ten months before kicking in your peaking phase. This will give you the fastest progress in developing total muscle mass. And as a side benefit you'll find it much easier to maintain a tight precontest diet when you know you'll blow an entire year of training if you don't reach optimum contest shape. At least that's the way it works for me."

### The Off-Season Cycle

The type of nutrition plan (chapter 5) and training program (chapter 6) already outlined are ideal for use during an off-season building cycle. The only difference is that you will train one weak muscle group with totally

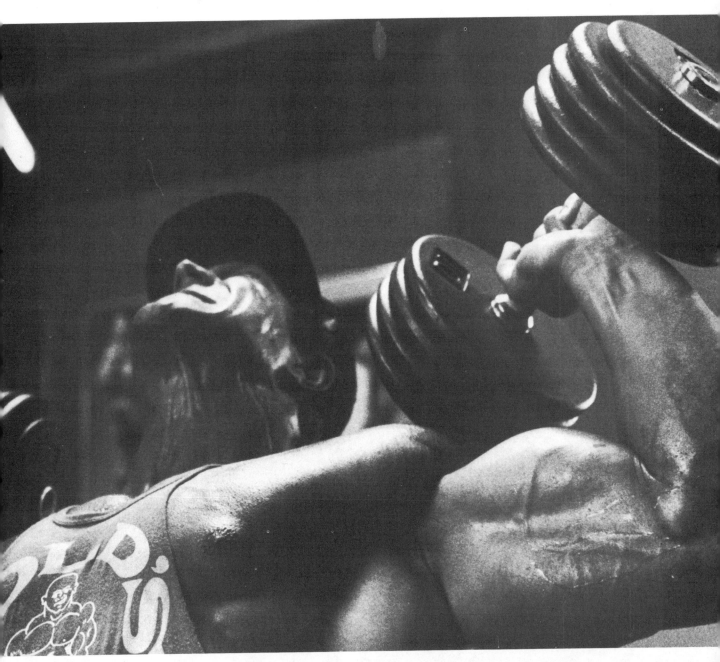

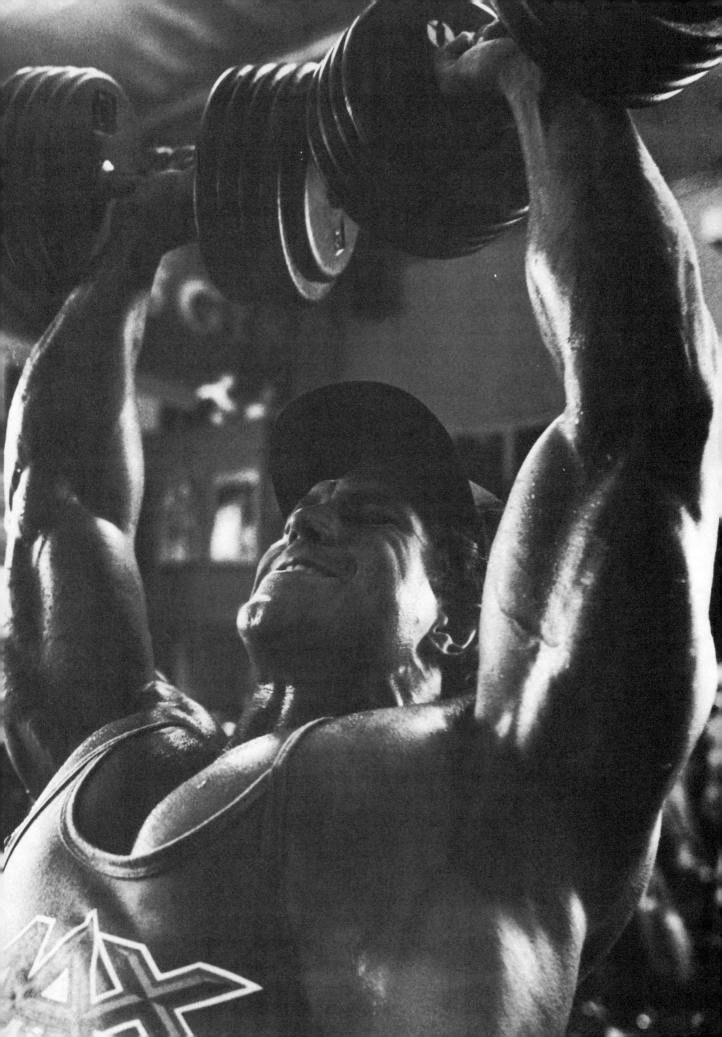

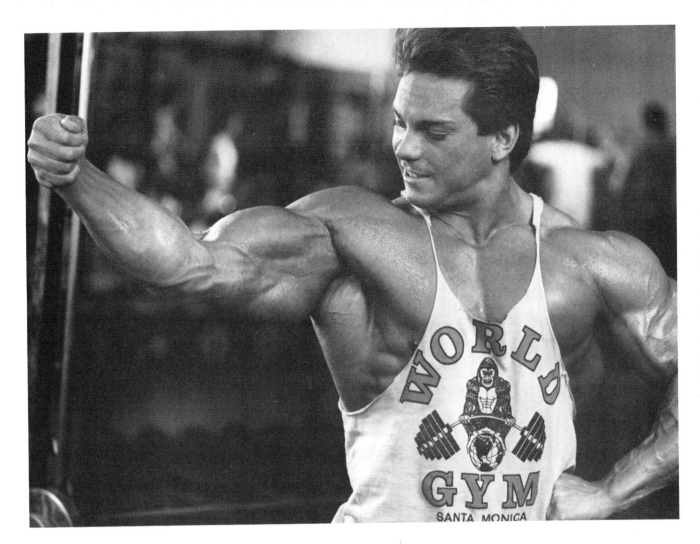

**Gaspari strikes a classic Larry Scott pose.**

awesome intensity off-season. But don't attempt to improve more than one weak point, because you'll only be able to reach top-level physical and mental intensity if you concentrate on specialized training for a single muscle group. However, you *can* rotate specialized training from one weak body part to another from month to month.

Many bodybuilders ignore aerobic training during the off-season, which I believe is a mistake. Thirty minutes of stationary cycling or fast walking three times per week will keep your aerobic conditioning level fairly high, maintaining cardiorespiratory and pulmonary fitness. And when a competition approaches you won't need to waste time breaking in to near-daily aerobic workouts.

### Transitional Cycles

Jumping directly from an off-season mode to a full precontest regimen from one day to the next would be a terrific shock to your body. In turn, this shock could make it difficult to maintain a contest diet and training routine. To a lesser extent, the same holds true if you abruptly switched from a precontest schedule to an off-season mode.

The solution to this problem is to schedule transitional cycles lasting two

**Heavy dumbbell presses.**

to three weeks between off-season and precontest cycles. In this way you can gradually break in to precontest training and dietary modes. Of course you will gradually intensify both training and diet right up to your show, but a transitional cycle keeps these changes from being so abrupt that they harm your body.

Let me give you an example. Let's say you normally work out four times per week and plan to follow a six-day split routine during a six-week peaking cycle. Over 1½ weeks you can gradually work up to five training sessions per day, then another 1½ weeks to gear up to the entire six-day-per-week program.

## The Precontest Cycle

You should refer to the chart (see Figure 1 on page 151) accompanying this section as you read about precontest training. But understand I'll be talking only about training. Refer to the *Gold's Gym Nutrition Bible* if you are unfamiliar with contest dieting.

The peaking procedure I usually recommend starts with two to three weeks on a four-day split, two to three more on a five-day split, two to three more on a six-day split (major muscle groups trained twice a week), two to three more on the six-day split in which you work major body parts three times per week, then finally three to four weeks on a double-split routine.

Parallel dips are one of the best exercises of all. Luiz Freitas, IFBB World Heavyweight Champion demonstrates them here. ➤

▼ The most frequently performed triceps exercise in the book is the pulley pushdown.

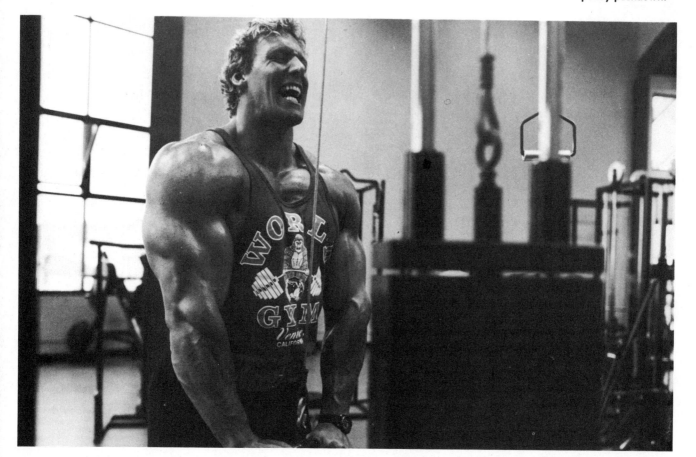

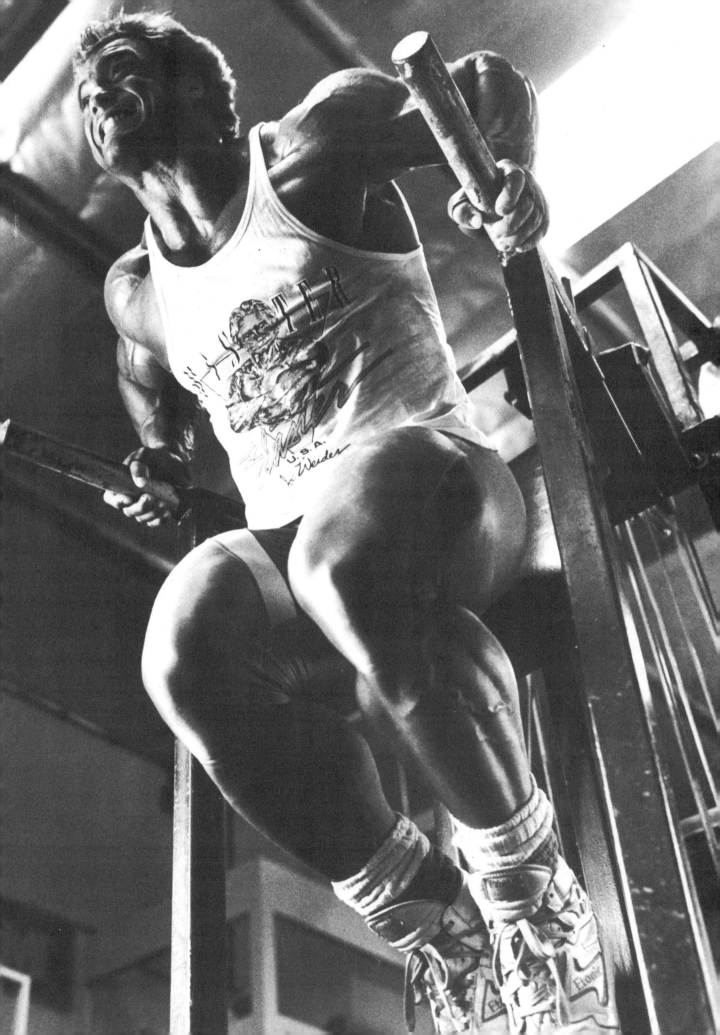

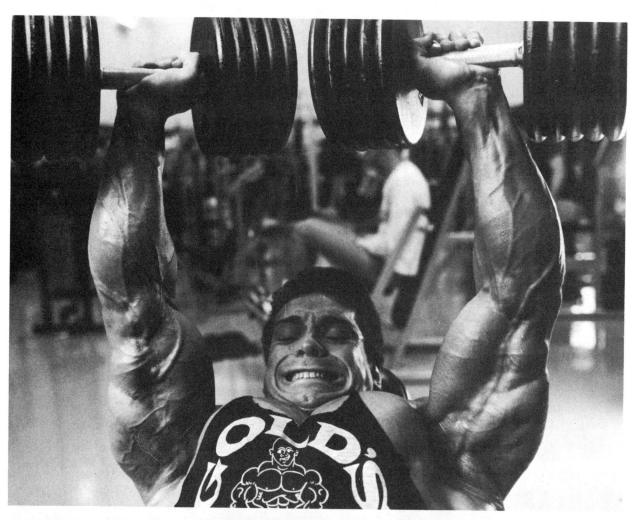

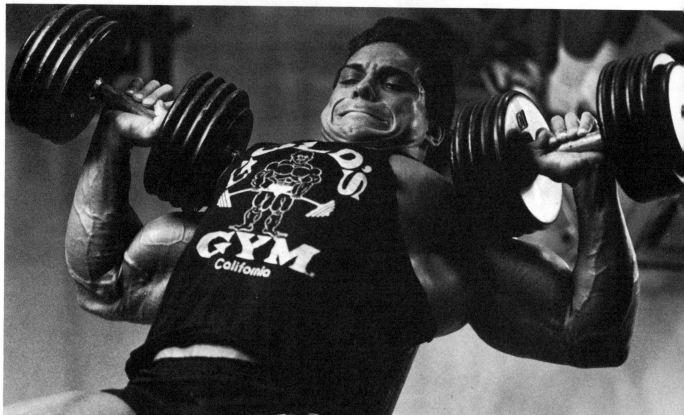

| Off-Season Cycle | Precontest Cycle |
|---|---|
| Four training days per week | Six training days per week |
| One workout per day | Often two weight workouts per day |
| Each major muscle group trained twice per week | Each major muscle group trained three times per week |
| Large muscle groups receive 10–12 total sets each workout, smaller body parts 6–8 | Large muscle groups receive 12–15 total sets each workout, smaller body parts 8–10 |
| Two or three minutes rest between sets | Thirty to sixty seconds rest between sets |
| Primary emphasis on basic exercises | Primary emphasis on isolation movements |
| Use of relatively low reps (5–8) each set | Use of high reps (10–15) each set |
| Emphasis on power training to build mass | Emphasis on muscularity workouts |
| Forced reps done on 1–2 sets per body part | Peak contraction and continuous tension on most sets |
| Three 30-minute aerobic sessions per week | Daily aerobic training, up to 1½–2 hours per day |
| Thirty minutes of posing practice three times per week | Daily posing practice, up to 1½–2 hours per day |

While you are gradually increasing the frequency of your workouts, you should also progressively increase the total sets done for each muscle group. Reps are also elevated while you gradually decrease the length of rest intervals between sets. You will become progressively more muscular with this type of program, combined with aerobic workouts and your tight precontest routine.

Aerobic training becomes increasingly important as a competition approaches, because it helps a bodybuilder achieve the leanest possible condition for each competition. While a heavy bodybuilding workout burns primarily glycogen (muscle sugar) to meet its energy needs, aerobic training actually burns stored body fat. The key to proper use of aerobics is to boost your heart rate up to at least 130–140 beats per minute, and then keep it there for at least 15 minutes.

The most popular forms of aerobic work prior to a competition are stationary cycling, ballistic cycling, fast walking, stair walking and running. A majority of champs will ride a stationary cycle 30–60 minutes per day, with some riding up to 2–3 hours daily. Many prefer to avoid running because they believe it wears muscle mass off of their upper bodies, particularly in the arms and shoulders.

"It's not at all uncommon," says pro champ Richie Gaspari, "for a serious competitive bodybuilder to do two weight workouts, one to two aerobic sessions and up to one hour of posing practice each day. It is advantageous to train several times per day when in a peaking mode, because every workout—whether aerobic or weight training—accelerates your metabolism for 1–2 hours after the session. Multiple workouts keep your BMR

◄ Gaspari uses terrific poundages on all his chest exercises.

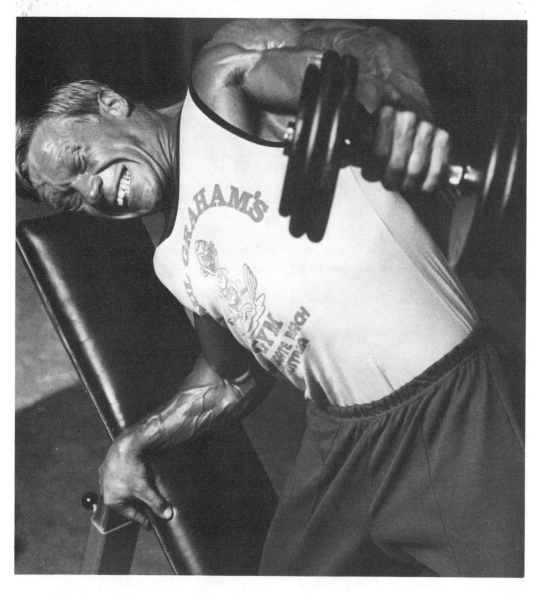

◄ One-arm side laterals are a terrific medial head developer.

up for a longer period each day than a single session, and that burns off body fat."

Lee Labrada (IFBB World Middleweight Champion and Pro Night of the Champions victor) continues: "Posing practice becomes extremely important as a competition approaches. Such practice not only helps you pose more smoothly and effectively, but also makes your physique appear harder and more muscular. I've found—like most serious bodybuilders—that the more posing practice I put in, the harder I look onstage."

Frank Zane agrees with Labrada. "When I was winning my Mr. Olympia titles," he reveals, "I practiced a routine in which I held each pose for 60 seconds, constantly trying to flex harder and bring out more detail as I held the pose. This was a key technique for muscle hardness, and it also gave me the ability to hold my poses relatively long without shaking like a leaf during prejudging comparisons."

There are two key training techniques—peak contraction and continuous tension—which also increase intramuscular detail for a competition. Robby

Robinson (Mr. America, Mr. World, Mr. Universe and victor at many IFBB pro shows) explains his use of these two techniques: "In peak contraction you should have a heavy weight on the fully contracted muscles at the top of the movement, which greatly increases tension in the muscles. While squats are not a peak contraction movement for quadriceps, leg extensions are great peak contraction work for quads. To enhance the peak contraction effect, I suggest holding the top position of the exercise for a slow count of two or three every repetition, attempting to almost cramp the muscles in this position.

"In continuous tension I attempt to slow down each rep and build extra tension into the working muscles, so I *feel* the entire repetition over its full range of motion. By also flexing the antagonistic muscles—for example, the triceps as you work biceps with barbell curls—you can actually use a relatively light weight and achieve the same effect as you can with heavier poundages in looser form.

"Prior to a competition, I use both peak contraction and continuous tension in all of my isolation exercises. I go for a burn in the working muscles every set before I allow myself to put the weight down. I give these two techniques plenty of credit for etching deep striations across every muscle group."

▼ Side laterals are the king of shoulder builders: Keijo Reiman.

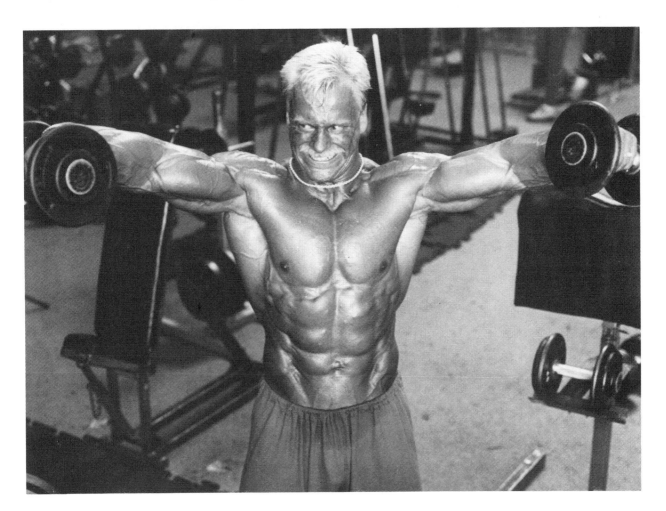

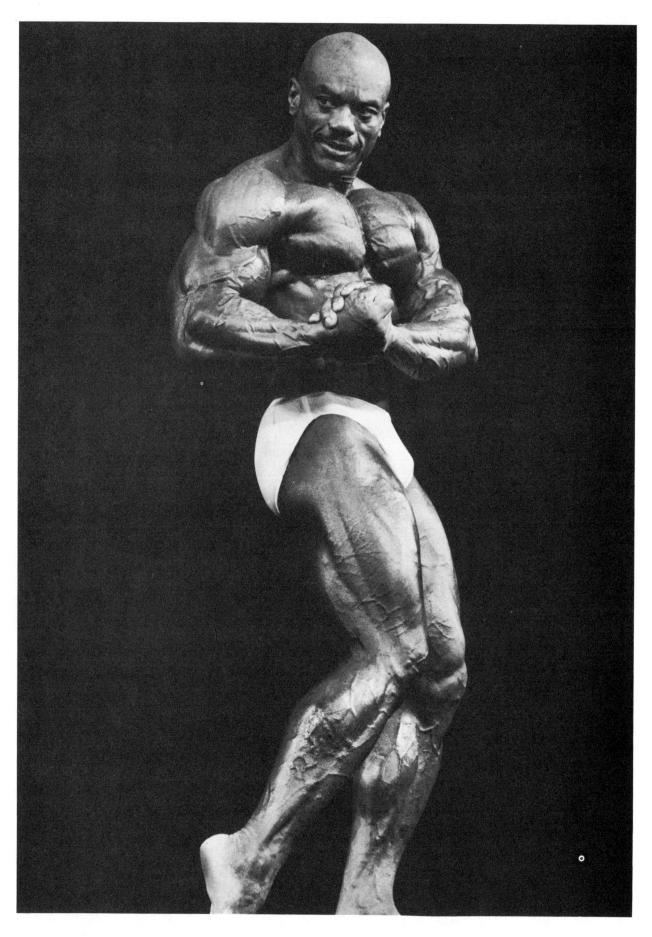

## Weak Point Specialization

"One avoidable problem in serious bodybuilding," says Lee Haney, "is that no two body parts will respond to hard work at exactly the same speed. Inevitably, some muscle groups forge ahead, gaining mass by leaps and bounds as a consequence of seemingly low-intensity effort in the gym. And just as inevitably, other body parts will lag behind in spite of seemingly Herculean efforts aimed at bringing them up to par with the remainder of the physique.

"One of the most fundamental qualities of a contest-winning physique is proportional balance, an equal development of every muscle group, with none visibly under- or overdeveloped. All the greats of the sport have almost ideally balanced proportions. And if you want to win some of the bigger titles, you absolutely must embark on a specialized training program that will help you to balance out your own physical proportions.

"I've been able to consistently bring my own weak points up through muscle priority training. In order to bring a lagging muscle group up to the level of the rest of your physique, you must train it with absolutely maximum intensity. The object is not to do longer and more involved workouts of twenty-five to thirty total sets. Instead, you must bomb the lagging body part with absolutely brutal intensity for a quick ten to twelve—perhaps up to fifteen if you're taking anabolics—total sets.

"It isn't easy to muster up this type of strength. You certainly can't expend such a huge amount of energy in so short a period of time toward the end of a workout, when your fuel tank is edging toward empty. It just stands to reason that such a high-intensity workout must take place at the beginning of a training session, when you have an absolute maximum amount of physical and mental energy available. And this is the essence of muscle priority training.

"Just as you schedule a weak muscle group first in your routine and bomb it with unmerciful intensity, you must also program your strongest body parts later in your training schedule and cut back on both the amount and intensity of work you give them.

"You should never worry about allowing a dominant muscle group to regress a little in development, because it will come up again very quickly with only eight to ten weeks of specialized work once the weaker area is improved. I've consistently priority-trained like this, and it has worked wonders for keeping my proportional balance as equal as it has been.

"In some cases, when a large muscle group needs improvement, muscle priority dictates that you train it by itself in a session. When I wanted to bring up my legs a couple of years ago, I did only legs two workout days out of every eight, dividing up the rest of my body parts into two equal sessions and bombing each part twice on four additional days. I also rested

◄ The one and only
Sergio Oliva.

completely two days out of every eight. This approach worked wonders for my legs."

In terms of training intensity when working on a lagging body part, Haney recommends following these eleven rules:

- Do fewer total sets than you normally would for a weak body part. I suggest reducing total sets by about 30 percent.
- Train fast. Even with the heaviest poundages, you should rest no more than about 90 seconds while working on large muscle groups, 60 seconds on smaller body parts.
- Attack each lagging muscle group from a maximum number of angles. A routine consisting of five sets each on two exercises is not as productive as one consisting of two sets each of five different movements.
- Psych up before each training session and stay highly motivated.

No one has deeper, thicker abs than Kawak. ➤

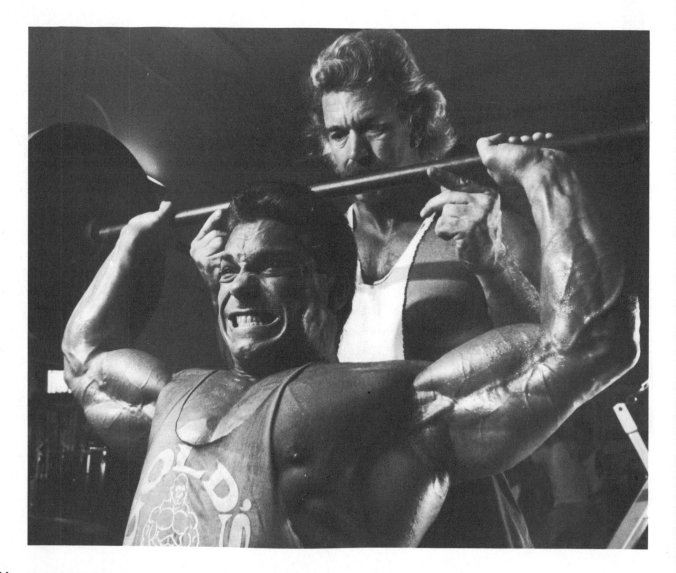

Rich Gaspari well into forced reps at Gold's Gym. Magic Schwartz assists.

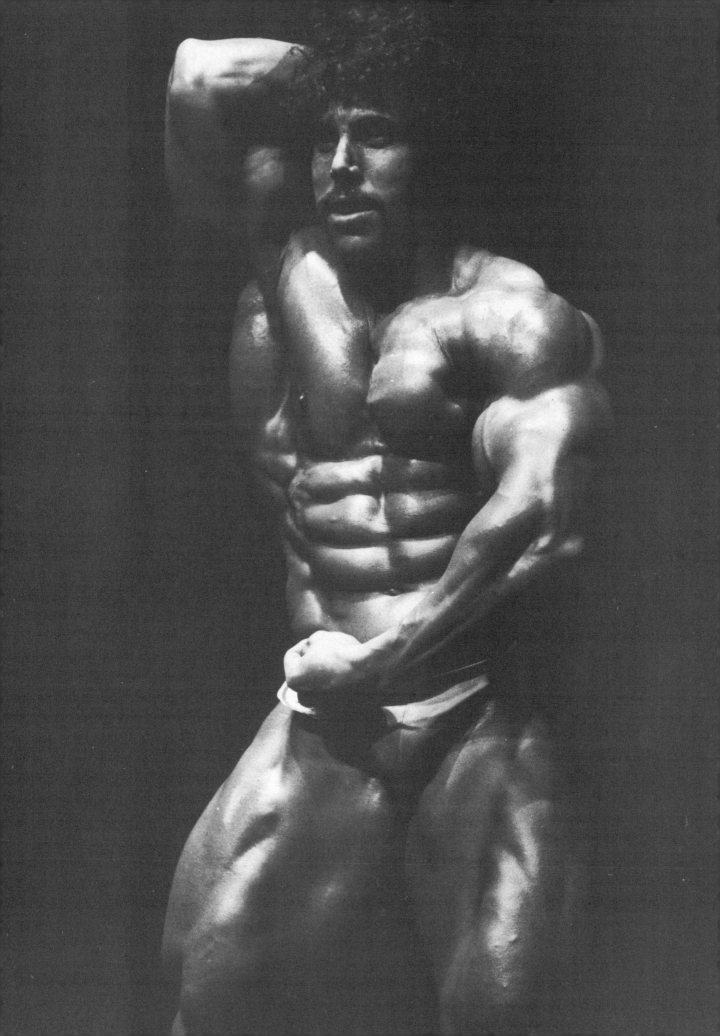

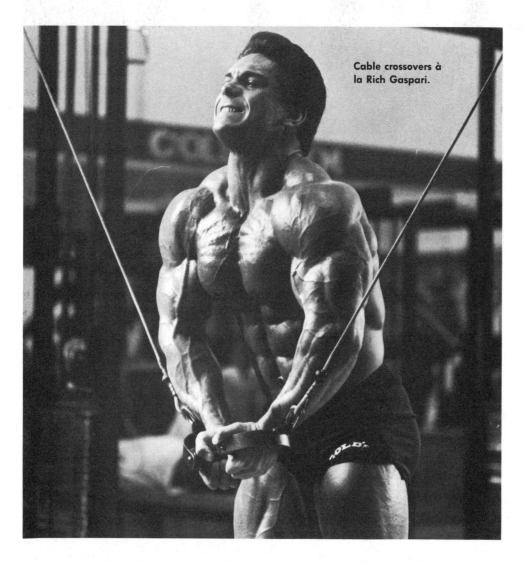

Cable crossovers à la Rich Gaspari.

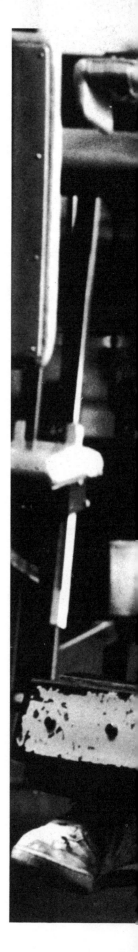

- Choose at least one heavy, basic exercise for the body part on which you are specializing and do at least two to three isolation movements for each muscle group in your specialization program.
- Use preexhaustion supersets when bombing lagging torso muscle groups such as pecs, delts, lats and traps.
- Use maximum poundages on each movement, following a thorough warm-up, but don't use so much weight on any one exercise that you are forced to sacrifice optimum body mechanics.
- Always maintain perfect form on every set of every exercise in your specialization program.
- Train at least to the point of failure on each post-warm-up set. And on many sets you can continue pushing well past the normal failure point by using forced reps.
- Make friends with pain. When going all out to improve a lagging muscle group, you will be constantly crashing past the

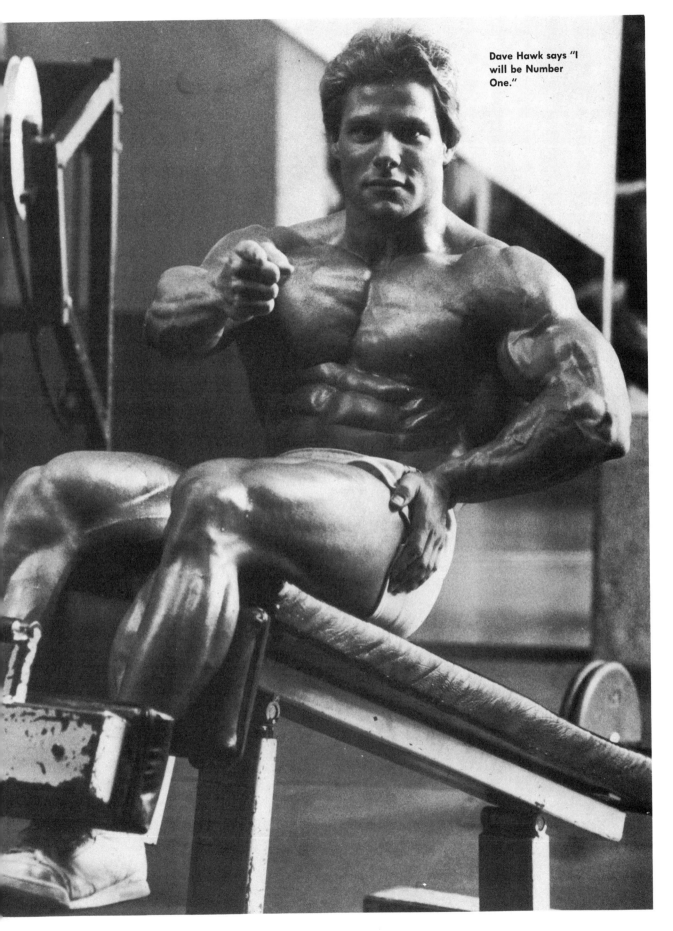

Dave Hawk says "I
will be Number
One."

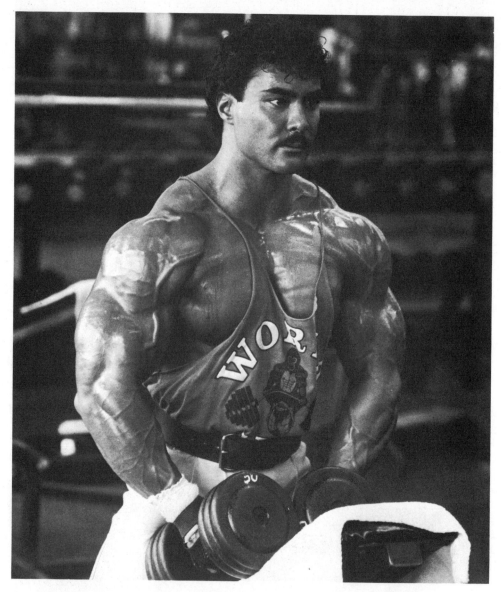

◄ Jon Aranita get-
ting psyched for a
heavy set of
dumbbell lateral
raises.

pain barrier. Rather than fearing this point in a set and therefore holding back a little on intensity, accept it as a sure
indication that you are training hard enough to induce muscle
hypertrophy.

- Maintain a positive mental attitude. You *will* improve, so get
into the gym and do it!

## Slowly, Slowly

One quality I've noticed in all champion bodybuilders is patience. They
know that Rome wasn't built in a day, and neither was any championship
physique. In reality, very few men have duplicated Arnold Schwarzenegger's
feat of winning his first Mr. Universe title after only five years of training.
Most men winning the smaller titles have three to five hard years of training
behind them. And most national contenders have eight to ten years of hard
training under their belts.

Renate Holland. ➤

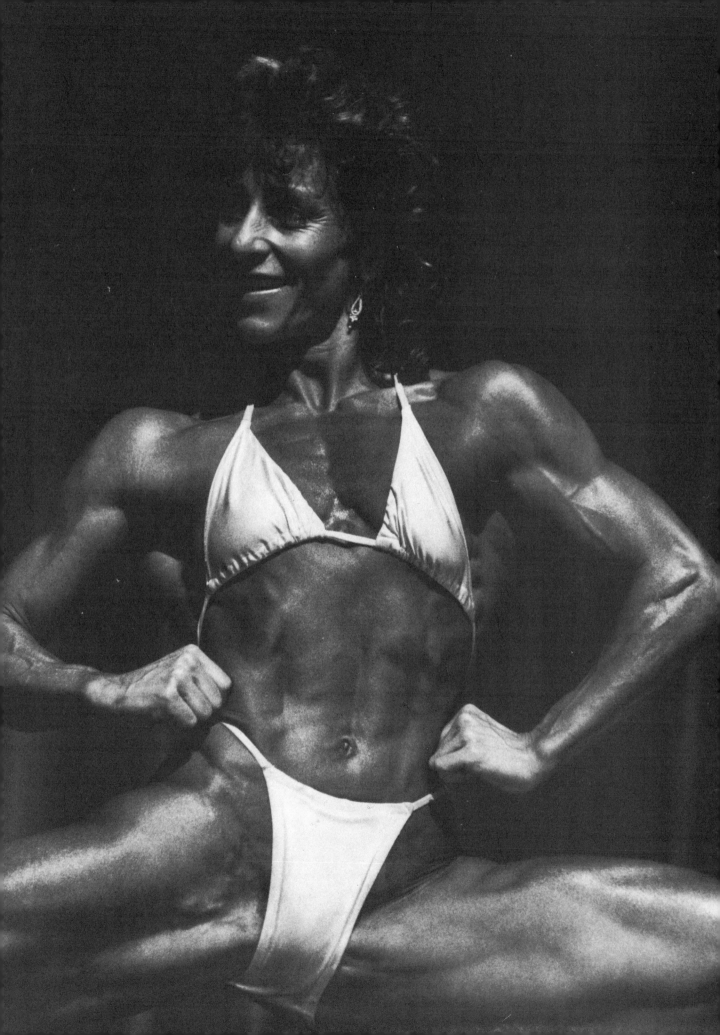

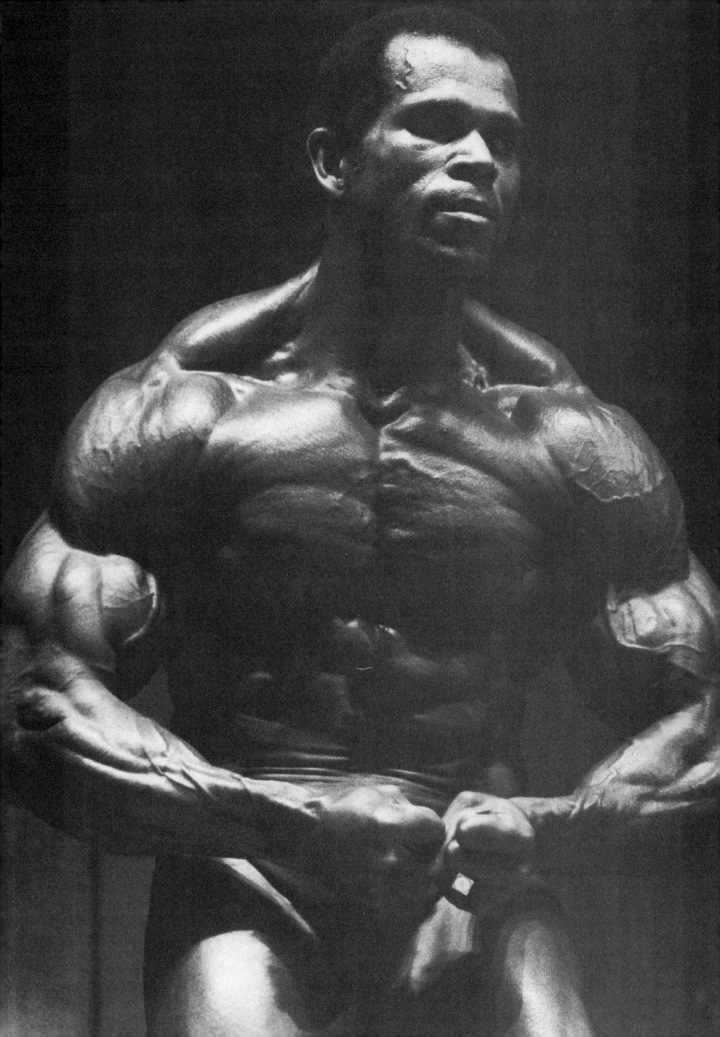

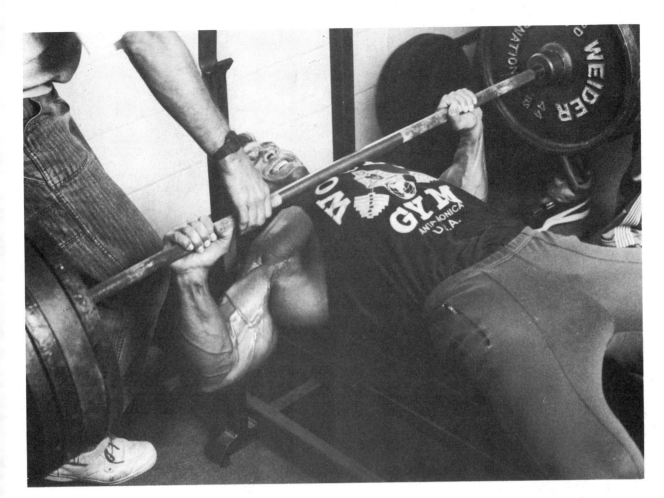

▲ Heavy benches are the mainstay of most chest routines.

◀ The superb pecs of the immortal Nubret.

Bodybuilders are more tortoises than hares. They keep grinding away week after week in the gym, celebrating even the smallest gains in muscle mass and quality. But step after step, gain after gain, the best bodybuilders develop terrific physiques. Even when they suffer competitive setbacks, they train hard and consistently.

You have a choice, so make the one that will ultimately make you a champion—make haste slowly.

### A Plea for Better Balance

As editor in chief of *Muscle & Fitness* for nearly ten years and editor in chief of *Flex* magazine since early 1987, I see one common mistake among rising competitive bodybuilders. Thinking they have awesome bodybuilding potential, they totally dedicate themselves to the sport, allowing the rest of their lives to drift off into oblivion. They neglect their education, job, family, everything but bodybuilding. I believe this is a giant mistake.

Shane DiMora (Teen, Junior and American National Champion at age 19) confesses, "I personally dedicated my life to bodybuilding at age 15, missing out on many of the normal teenage experiences. I couldn't even go to see a film because it interfered with my nutrition schedule, and I couldn't miss meals and succeed as a bodybuilder. School was ranked a

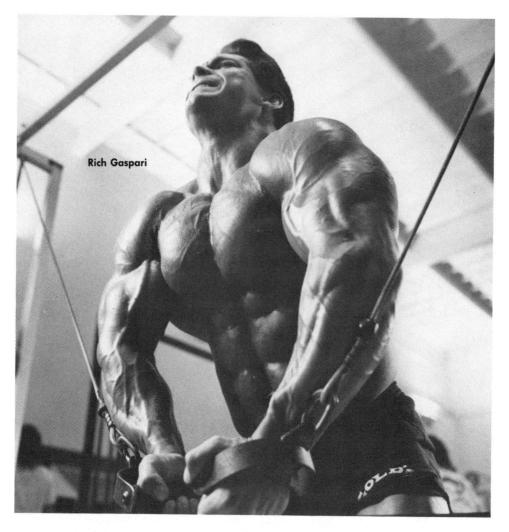

Rich Gaspari

distant second to bodybuilding, and my social life was abbreviated compared to my friends'.

"If I had it to do again, I'd have at least finished high school before getting serious. That might have meant winning Nationals and turning pro at 20 instead of 19, but I'd be much better rounded now than I am. So in all of my training seminars I tell young bodybuilders to finish school and get a good job before getting totally dedicated to bodybuilding.

"It's a shame to see how many young guys with little potential for the sport decide to be pros at an early age. They end up winning only small shows—perhaps even no shows—and are washed up with no schooling, no job, and alienated friends and relatives when they are 30 or 35. It's much better to take your time and develop a support system, and then go for the gold."

Tom Platz says, "Stop and smell the flowers as you rise in the sport. All of the top guys—my personal friends—are tremendously well-rounded individuals. In my opinion, you can't become a bodybuilding superstar without also being a well-rounded, well-educated person. Yes, stop and smell the flowers."

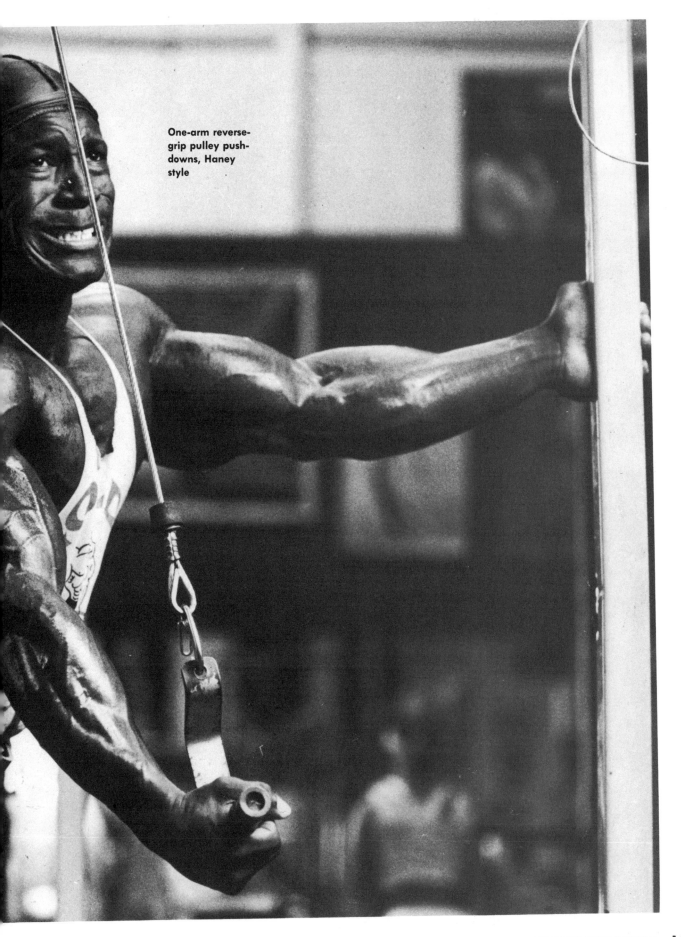

One-arm reverse-grip pulley push-downs, Haney style

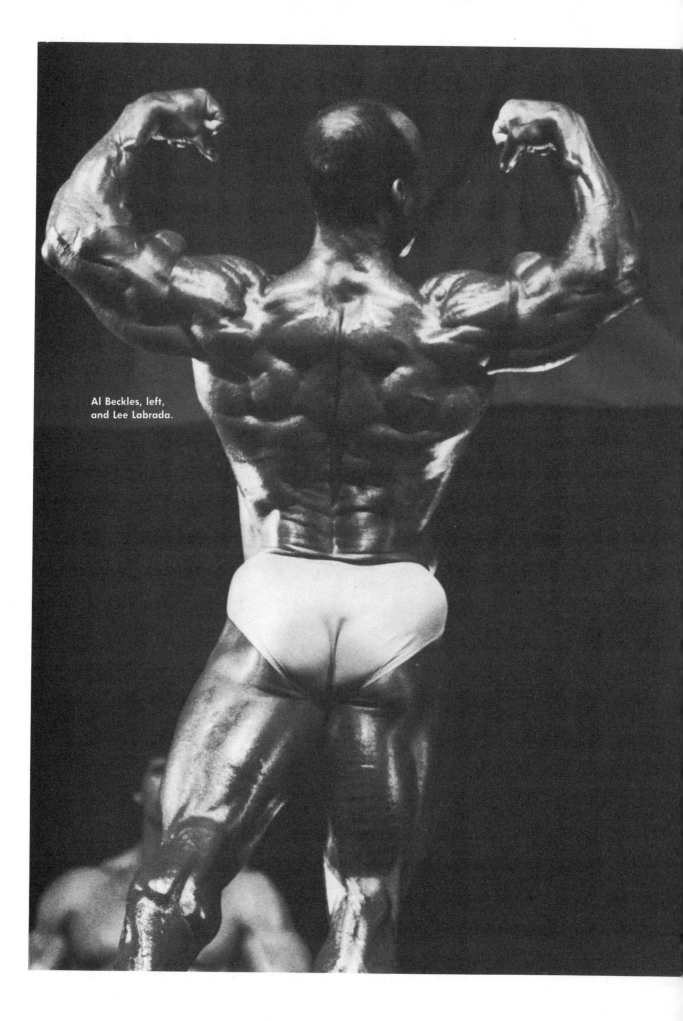

Al Beckles, left,
and Lee Labrada.

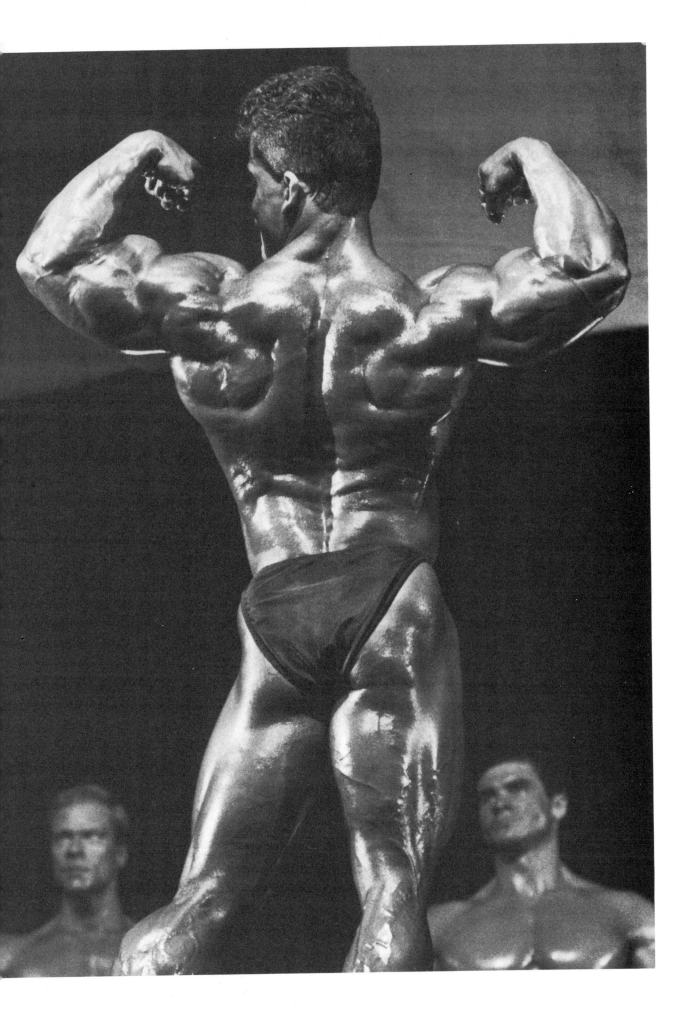

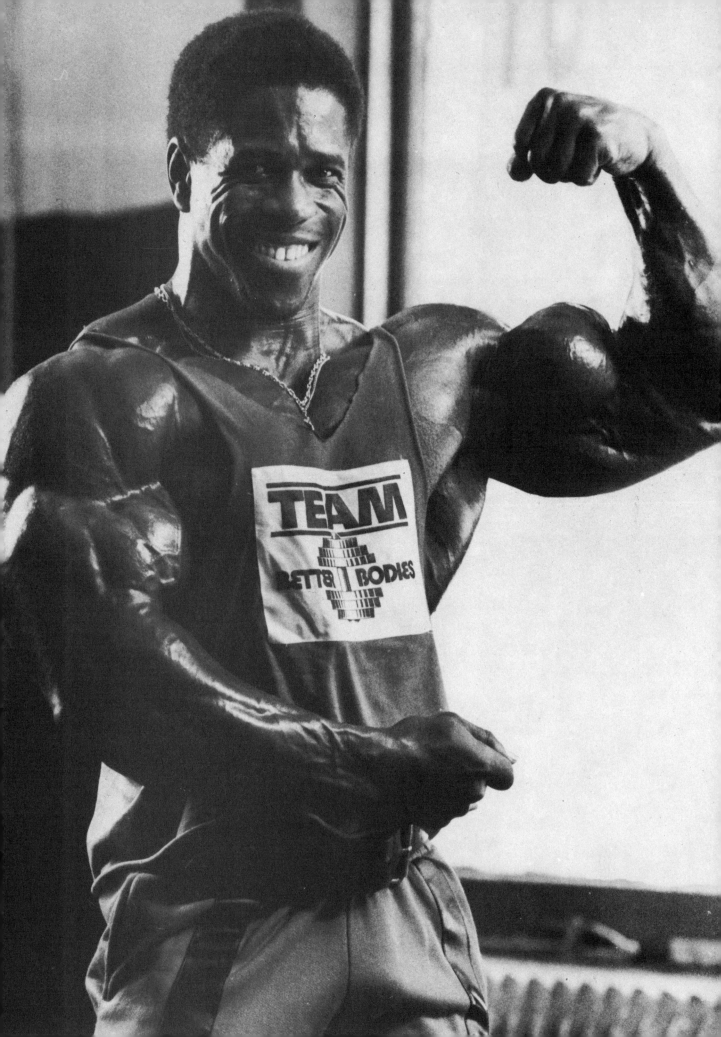

# 8

# Freestyle Bodybuilding

The ultimate aim of every freestyle bodybuilder should be to develop reliable instincts for what his or her body requires each day in terms of workout load and nutrition in order to continue making optimum gains. All of the most successful athletes in the sport have developed their innate training and dietary instincts.

I'll let the coverman of this book, Lee Labrada, give you his personal viewpoint on instinctive training ability: "There are two levels of instinctive training ability, a basic type which helps you to tell as quickly as possible whether or not a new training or dietary variable is working well for your unique physique; and a higher level which allows your body to tell your mind precisely what it needs to be given in terms of training and nutrition variables in order to keep increasing in muscle mass and quality.

"Without this first type of instinctive training ability, you would waste months, perhaps years, in going down dead-end alleys as you search for the precise workout factors and dietary variables which allow you to gain muscle quickly and efficiently. The essence of bodybuilding is the experiment. You must use your body as a sort of laboratory in which you conduct

◀ Bertil Fox.

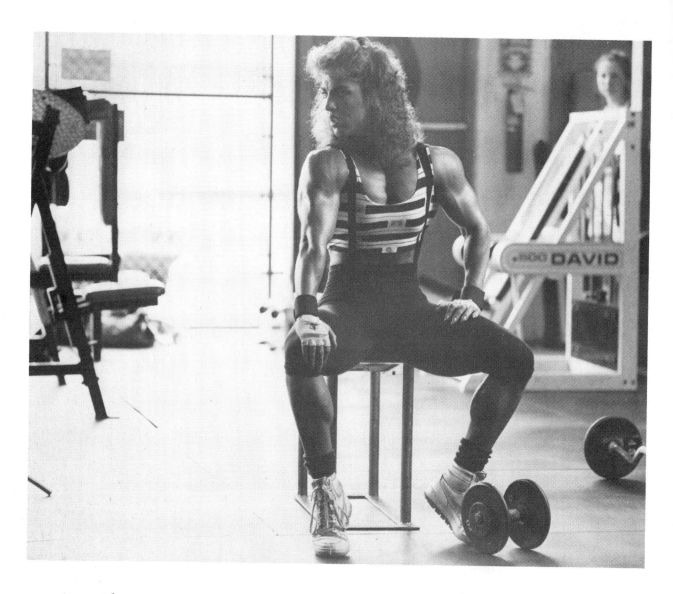

experiment after experiment to determine which exercises, set-rep schemes, training tempos, and other factors result in the quickest possible gains in muscle mass.

"Over a period of time, you will spend a couple of weeks or months doing sets of five to six reps for a particular muscle group, a few more doing seven to eight reps, more doing nine to ten, and so forth up to perhaps twenty reps. By monitoring the biofeedback data your body gives you during each of these experiments, you can easily and quickly determine which repetition patterns work best for your unique body and physiological system.

"Within a couple of years, you will become so good at interpreting the biofeedback your body sends back to your mind, you will reach the second level of instinctive training ability—the ability to determine each day precisely what your body needs in terms of training and nutrition in order to continue growing optimally. Most bodybuilders can reach this point if they try to, but many don't make the effort. While some general training var-

▲ Cathey Palyo at Gold's Gym, April 1987.

Mike Quinn tortures his delts during intense sets of machine side laterals. ▶

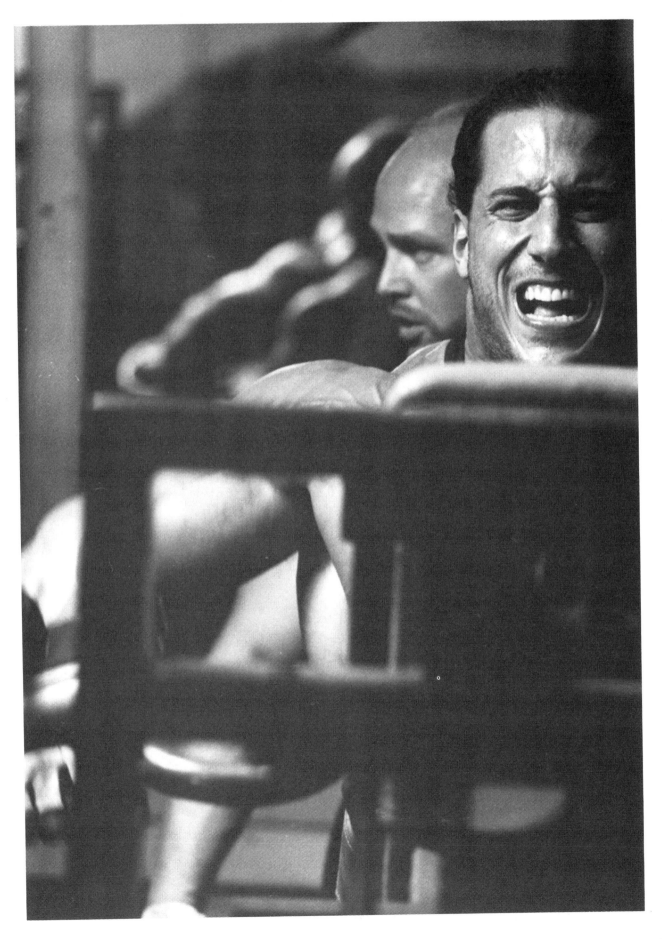

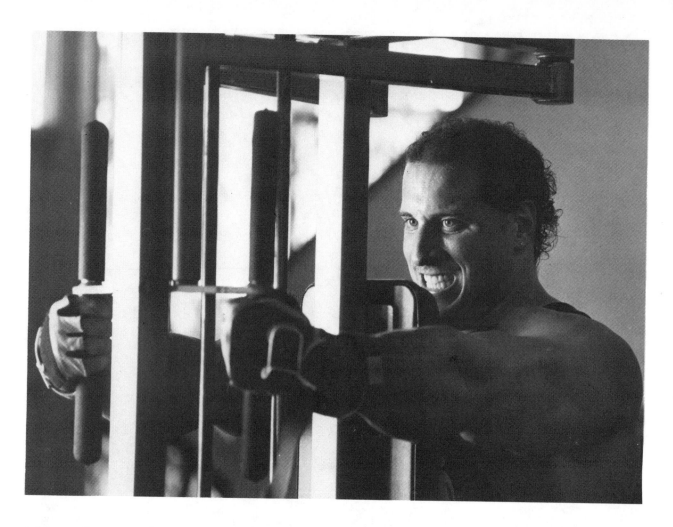

Rear delt laterals on the machine.

iables will work well each workout day, you will always be faced with facets of your training which can be interpreted and performed in a variety of ways. When you are able to interpret each of these variables accurately, you will have reached the second level of training instinct, and you'll be making the fastest gains of your bodybuilding career."

For the first few months a bodybuilder is steadily training, he should follow a set routine and not attempt to determine which training and nutritional variables work best for him. It takes several months of steady training on a basic routine to build up a familiarity with the activity, plus develop sufficient strength to push workouts hard enough to make gains past the intermediate level of the sport.

You won't be able to follow someone else's routine for more than five to six months, however. While all bodies respond to specific general stimuli, there are hundreds of subvariables that govern how well a bodybuilder will progress at the more advanced levels of the sport. Even a casual inspection of some of the training articles you might see in *Flex* magazine will convince you that every bodybuilder trains and eats in a uniquely personal way.

"Learn to listen to your body," says IFBB pro bodybuilder Tony Pearson (Mr. America, Mr. World and Mr. Universe). "It talks to you constantly,

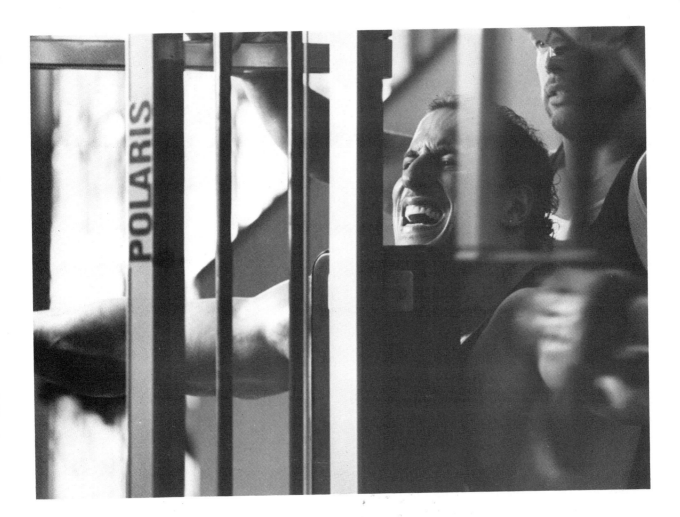

and you have to learn to listen to what it is telling you. If you adopt the policy of constantly listening to what your body says to you—and interpreting what it says about what you should be doing to help it make muscle-mass gains—you'll make excellent long-term gains as a bodybuilder."

As I've written before (in *The Gold's Gym Book of Bodybuilding*), "These signals can be as obvious as a great muscle pump from a particular set or as a good psychological response to a new training technique.

"Muscle pump is probably the biofeedback signal that most bodybuilders monitor. Around Gold's Gym you constantly hear Lou Ferrigno or someone else saying, 'Wow, I really got a good pump in my biceps with the routine I'm on!' And a good pump—a tight, blood-congested feeling in a muscle— is a reliable signal that you've trained a particular muscle group optimally."

Muscle soreness after a particularly stiff workout is also a good indication that you are on the right track in your training. As Lou Ferrigno (Teenage Mr. America, Mr. America, Mr. International and twice IFBB Mr. Universe) says, "You want your muscles to be a little stiff and sore to the touch, but having very sore muscles a day after training means you've pushed too hard in a workout. Press your fingers into a muscle to test how sore it is. If you feel sharp pain, your muscles are too sore. If the pain is mild and

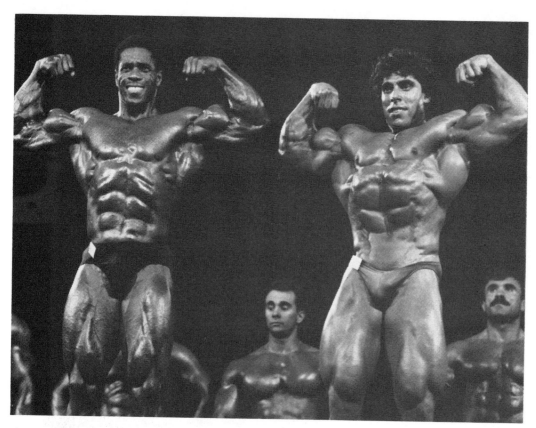

▲ Fox and Kawak at the 1987 New York Night of Champions.

almost pleasurable, you have gotten a great workout for that particular body part, and you should stick to it for a while.

"The secret to bodybuilding in general, and to instinctive training in particular, is a willingness to learn from experience. Sure, it's good to go for a full pump in each working muscle group, but pushing past this point is deleterious to the muscles. If you go too far in a workout, you'll lose your pump, a sure sign that you've done too much. Do just enough to achieve a maximum pump in each muscle group, and then move on to work your next body part.

"A deep growth burn in the muscles is another positive biofeedback signal that your body will send you. Going for this burn every workout guarantees you a maximum growth stimulus from a workout. Try to feel a maximum growth burn on only the final set or two of each exercise, however. Going too deeply into a growth burn can turn off your mind and body to training. For some bodybuilders, it's just too painful to go for a deep burn on every set!"

As you become more experienced in bodybuilding, you will learn to crash past this pain barrier in your workouts. When you burst the pain barrier frequently enough in your workout, you force your muscles to grow large and strong, larger and stronger than is possible without punching past this pain barrier. But this is a very advanced technique applicable

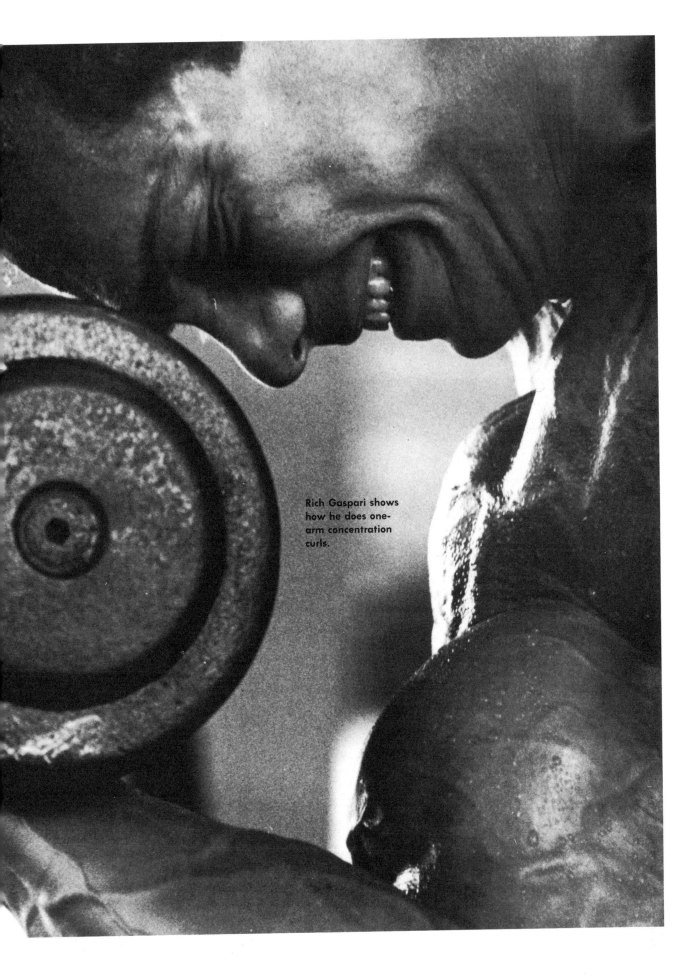

Rich Gaspari shows how he does one-arm concentration curls.

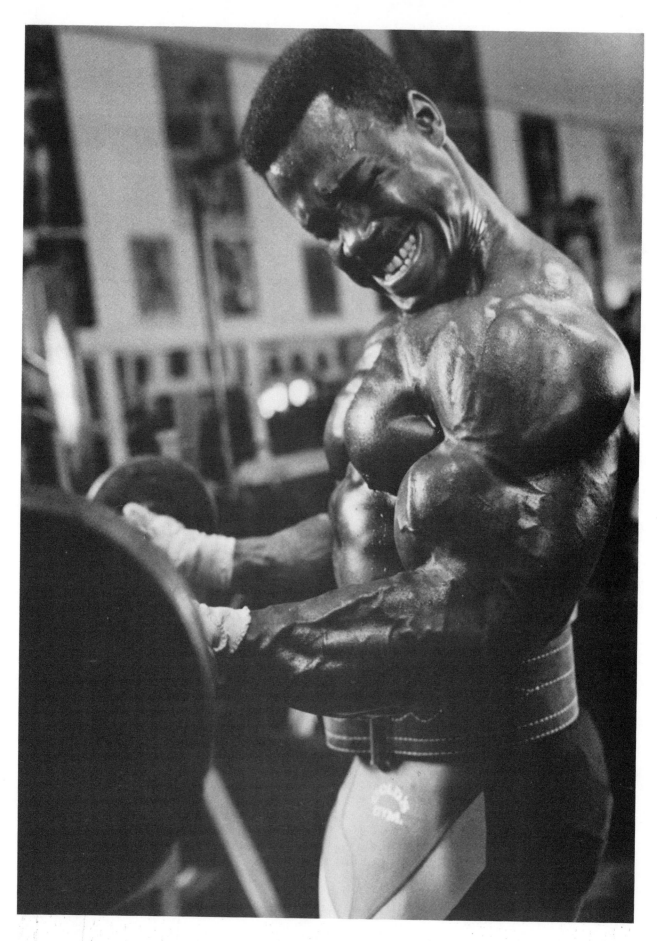

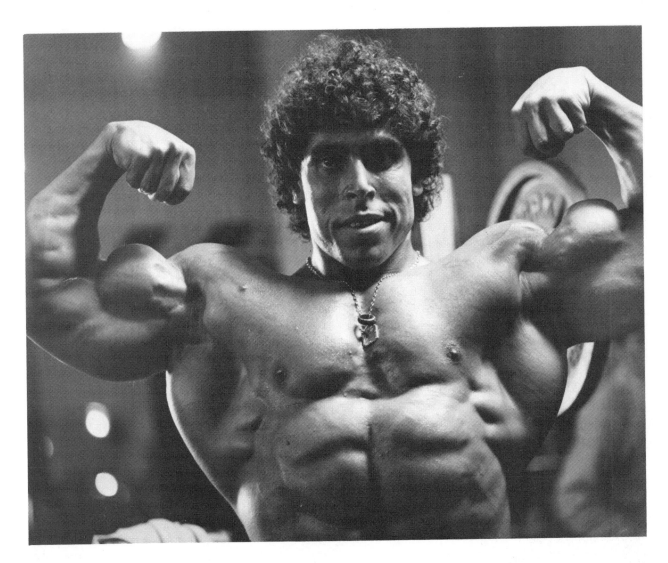

▲ Kawak's amazing body.

◀ Dumbbell curls: Michael Ashley.

primarily to bodybuilders on the verge of entering a competition, or already experienced competitors.

Growth pain and pump are just two of several internal muscular sensations that you should be monitoring. Some others are the intensity of each muscular contraction, feelings of great energy or residual fatigue, soreness in joints and connective tissues, and a general feeling of power and workout momentum.

"One of the most obvious biofeedback signals you should be monitoring," says Lee Haney, "is how quickly or slowly you are making gains in strength on each exercise in your routine. At the lower levels of the sport—up to the point where you have been training at least two to three years—there is a direct correlation between your strength for several reps in good form on a particular basic exercise and the mass and quality of those muscles which move the weight in that exercise.

"Therefore, you should definitely monitor your increasing strength levels. The easiest way to do this is to maintain a training diary in which you record each day every exercise you perform, the amount of weight you used for each set, and the number of repetitions you did with this weight every set. You can either use a commercially prepared training diary, or simply make notes in any bound notebook. A lot of bodybuilders like to use account ledgers, which are bound like a normal hardback book. They can be found in any business supplies store.

"One problem with monitoring increases in training poundages is that it's difficult to see changes from one workout to the next, or from one week to the next, for that matter. This is where a well-maintained training diary comes into play. You can look back a month, six months, a year, even longer, and you can graphically *see* upward trends in training poundages which are quite large in magnitude. And when you see such great increases in the weights you have been handling, your enthusiasm for your workouts will soar. Even if you haven't noticed a gain in a couple of months on a particular exercise, you can see that you've gained more than 75 pounds on that movement since you started bodybuilding, and you go into the gym for your next workout charged up to make the same type of gains in the following couple of years."

By keeping a photographic record of your progress in your training diary, you can also see your progress from one month—or one year—to the next. The best way to do this is to have Polaroids taken of your physique in standard poses (front and back double biceps, front and back lat spreads,

The amazing biceps of Britain's Bertil Fox. ➤

▼ Greg Comeaux checks out the impressive biceps of Mr. USA Mike Quinn.

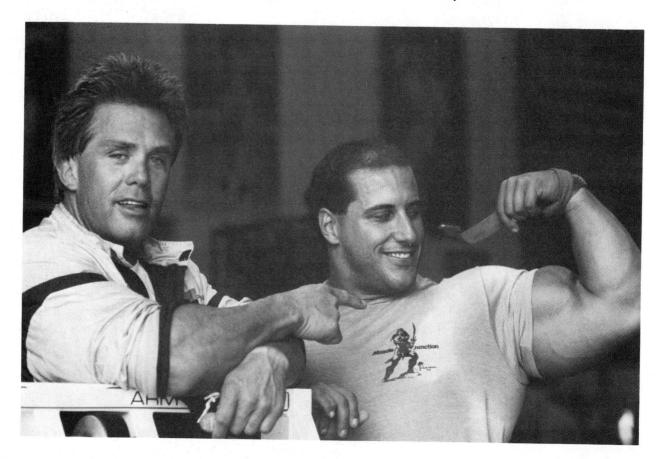

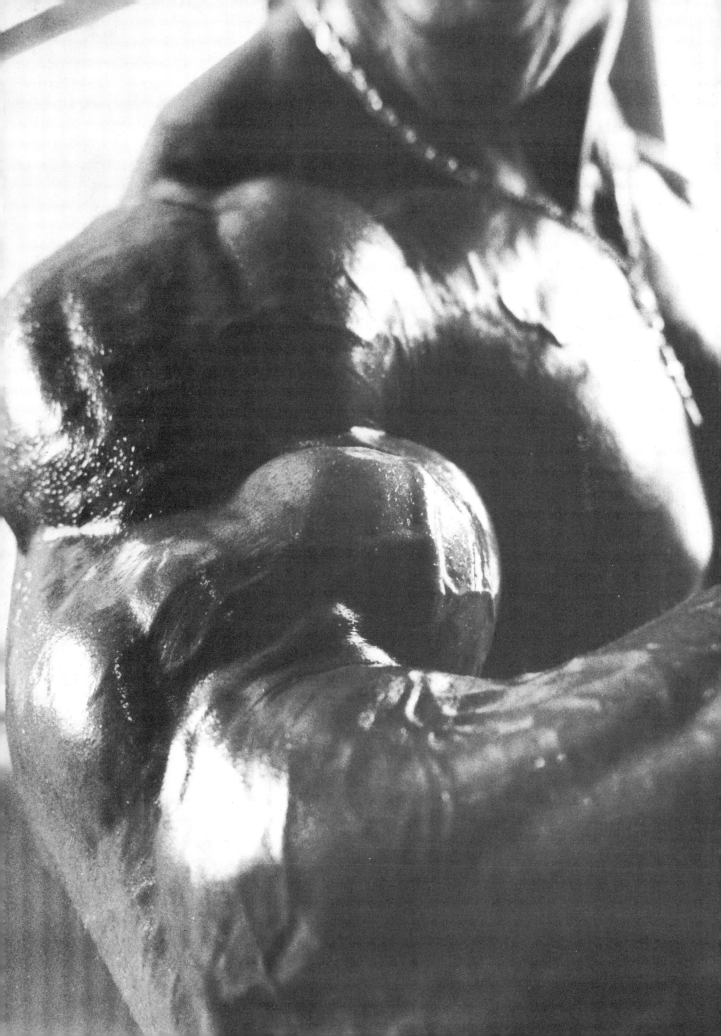

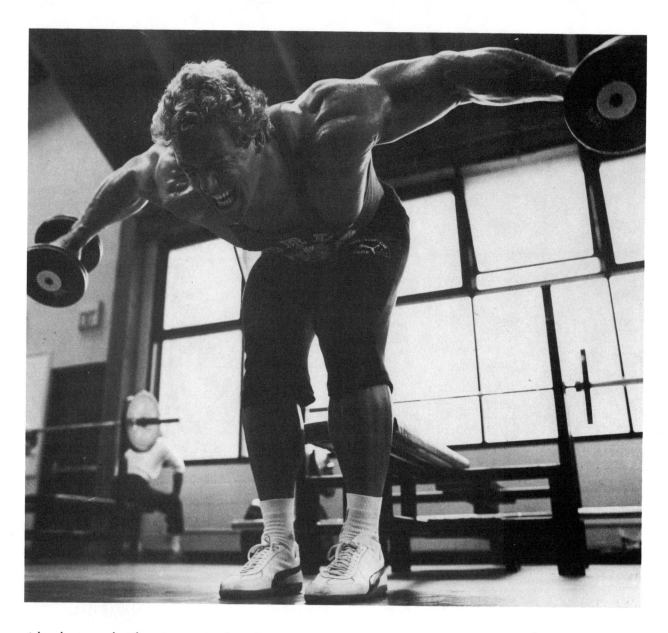

side chest and side triceps, and perhaps a most muscular shot) each four to six weeks. Paste them in your diary, and refer back to them periodically.

During your first few weeks of training, you can actually see improvement in your physique from one day to the next. Certainly, you can see improvement from one week to the next. But as time passes, it becomes harder and harder to see such improvements in your body. So when you become discouraged that you aren't making any progress, check back in your diary for photos taken three, six or twelve months ago, and you'll graphically see progress. And you'll know that you're on the right track instinctively, that you've instinctively learned which exercises, routines, training techniques and nutritional variables work best for your unique body and physiological system.

"Measurements are a good way to determine if you are making gains at the beginning and intermediate levels," reveals Mike Christian (National

▲ **Ralf Moeller trains all three heads of the deltoid muscle.**

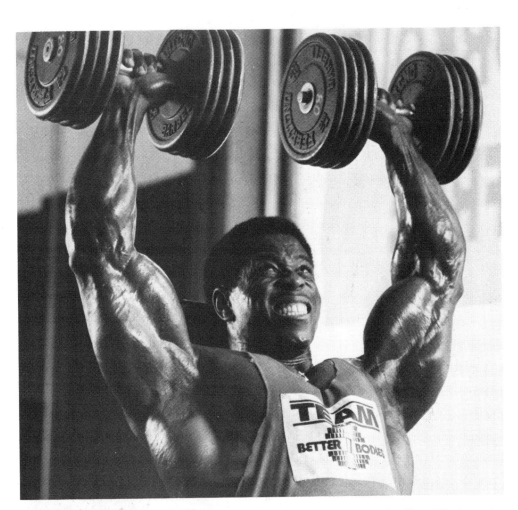

Heavy dumbbell presses have been one of Fox's favorite exercises for over twenty years.

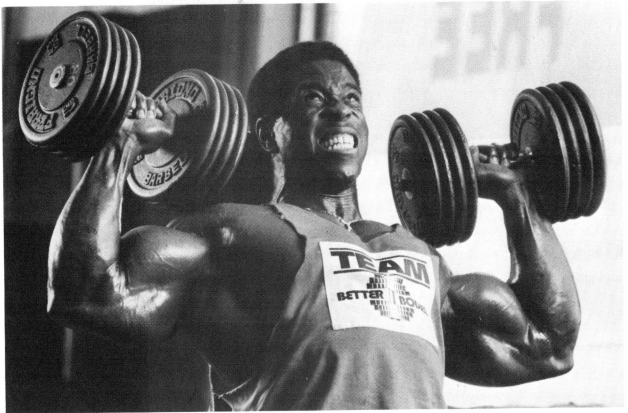

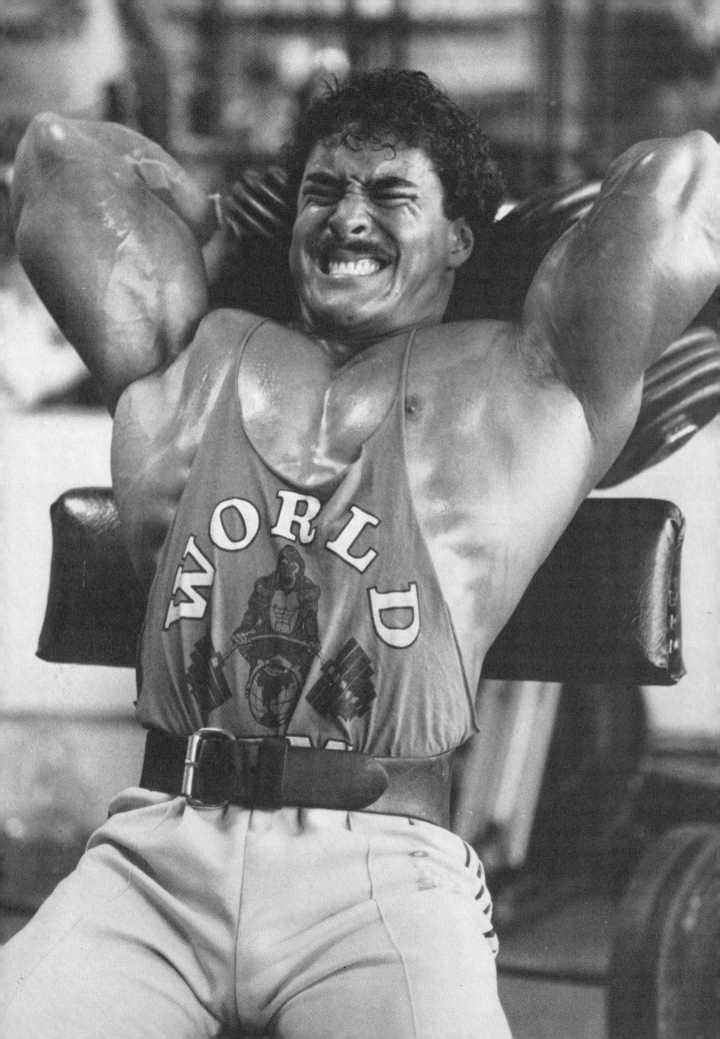

and World Heavyweight Champion, and a professional bodybuilder who has placed as high as third in Mr. Olympia). "But in order for these measurements to be of comparative value to you, they must be taken under standardized conditions. That means when your muscles are cold—not warmed up—as they are when you get up in the morning after a night's sleep. Simply measure the girth of your expanded chest, flexed upper arm, forearm, waist, thigh and calf.

"Past the first ten to twelve months of bodybuilding, measurements will cease to be of value to you, because you won't be making gains at the same fast pace you did in the first weeks of your bodybuilding training experience. Also for advanced bodybuilders measurements are relatively worthless because they don't gauge the quality of a particular muscle group, only its relative mass. Quality is far more important than mere mass to a competitive bodybuilder. Competitors are much better off compiling visual evidence of their gains, which means having photos taken at regular intervals in standard poses."

As I wrote in the *Gold's Gym Book of Bodybuilding*, "There are tactile and visual factors that can also improve your training instinct. You can test your muscle density—hardness—simply by feeling each muscle group with your hand from time to time. Greater muscle density indicates that your training and dietary techniques are successful. It's also easy to see improvements in your physique in various poses in front of a mirror."

Following are several more biofeedback variables that you should monitor in your efforts to gradually learn an instinctive, freestyle approach to your bodybuilding:

- Lack or presence of enthusiasm for workouts
- Relative sense of motor coordination
- Sensations of excessive stress, or lack of stress
- Feelings of energy depletion
- Irritability
- Soreness, stiffness, slowness to get warmed up
- Hunger
- Steady or elevated morning pulse rate
- Steady or elevated morning blood pressure

Frank Zane feels you should also consider subconscious sources of biofeedback: "Successful bodybuilding depends on expansion of awareness into particular areas. A great deal of information is being fed to you unconsciously. You receive clues from the subconscious mind all of the time, and a bodybuilder who shuts off his unconscious mind to live only in the conscious side of his life misses more than half of the input he *could* receive.

◄ Jon Aranita doing two-dumbbell seated triceps extensions. Jon uses up to 70-pound dumbbells on this exercise.

The unconscious mind is the source of all creativity. If you disregard this in your mental approach to bodybuilding, you will not develop a unique physique. Remain open for ways to improve your physique. Don't feel that you know everything there is to know about bodybuilding and get locked up in your own ego."

Joe Weider (publisher of *Flex* and *Muscle & Fitness* magazines) continues: "There are several ways in which you can open your mind to unconscious feedback signals. Initially, you need only resolve to maintain an open mind, which will in turn open up your conscious mind to stimuli it would never notice otherwise. Later, you can use hypnosis and various meditation techniques to further reveal the subconscious biofeedback signals that you would normally fail to recognize.

"Implicit in use of the instinctive training principle in evaluating various training techniques, exercises and routines is a thorough knowledge of bodybuilding training and nutrition. You should read every book and magazine on bodybuilding and related sports you can collect in an effort to further advance your knowledge of the sport.

"I also firmly believe that you should carefully study science and technical books which might include information that has a bearing on your approach to bodybuilding. Some of the subjects that you should study are anatomy, kinesiology, biomechanics, exercise physiology, biochemistry and psychology. You might even consider taking college classes either part- or full-time in an effort to learn more about the scientific principles underlying muscle growth."

According to Boyer Coe (Mr. America, many times Mr. Universe, Mr. World and an IFBB World Pro Grand Prix Champion), it's easier to determine which nutritional variables work best than it is to decide on the best training factors: "As in developing a training philosophy, this involves trying every possible food element in your diet for a couple of weeks at a time to decide if, and how well, it works for you. But where it might take six to eight weeks to tell if preexhaustion supersets work well for you, it might take only a few days to determine if inosine is a valuable nutrient for your bodybuilding efforts.

"During a two- or three-week trial with a food element, you can monitor your body's biofeedback to determine what effect that food or supplement has had on your body. As an example, if you ate a pint of pistachio ice

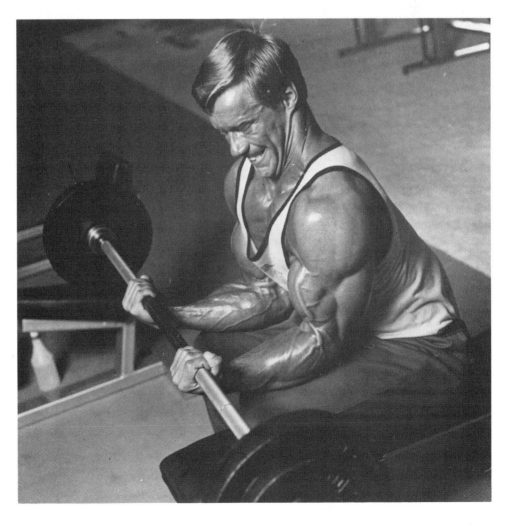

Seated wrist curls are the most direct forearm exercise known: Jyrki Saavolanen.

cream every day for three weeks, a certain piece of biofeedback data—the fact that you're growing incredibly fat—will tell you that food's effect on your body.

"Try to decide if a new food element gives you greater workout energy. Does it allow you to sleep better and recuperate more completely? Does it make your skin healthier looking? Does it help to define you before a show, or does it prevent you from achieving maximum muscular definition? How does it affect your range of emotions? By monitoring all of the bio-feedback that your body eventually provides you, you can develop an instinct for how a training or dietary factor is working in your body. Instinctive training ability—both in training and diet—is one of the most valuable skills any bodybuilder can develop."

Joe Weider continues: "Once mastered, the instinctive principle allows you to be in harmony with the natural up and down energy cycles through which your body goes. No one feels highly energetic very frequently, but when you *are* bursting with energy you should take advantage of it by training long, hard and heavy. But pushing this hard when you are on an energy downswing will result in a progress-slowing injury or an overtrained condition in which it becomes impossible to make gains, no matter how hard or consistently you train.

"If your instinctive training ability has been finely honed, you will be able to easily identify your up and down days, matching the intensity of your workouts to sync with your energy levels. This way, you will always train as intensely as possible, but still far enough within your abilities that you can avoid injuries and the chance of overtraining."

Powerful Richard Gaspari (National and World Light Heavyweight Champion, victor in many IFBB pro shows, and a man who has twice placed second in Mr. Olympia) tells how he trains instinctively from one workout to another: "When I go into the gym I know which muscle groups I'll be training and what my first exercise will be for each body part, but I don't know what routine I will follow, how heavy I'll go and which training intensification techniques I'll use. But during my first two to three sets of my warm-up for each muscle group, I can automatically tell how much energy I have and even what type of training program I should follow in order to stimulate maximum muscle hypertrophy.

"Throughout my workout I'll constantly update my impressions of what my body is telling me to do. I'll gain a clearer and clearer picture of what my body requires in each workout as I get further into that day's training schedule. This way I can push my body instinctively to its maximum for that one workout day without pushing past that fine line between optimum intensity and overtraining. That way my instinctive training ability allows me to make optimum gains from my workouts and dietary efforts."

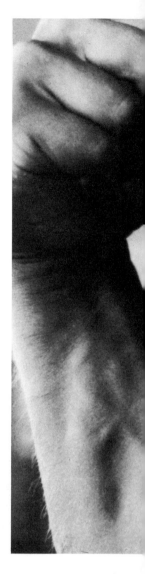

Mike Quinn proba- ▲ bly has the most impressive arms in bodybuilding today.

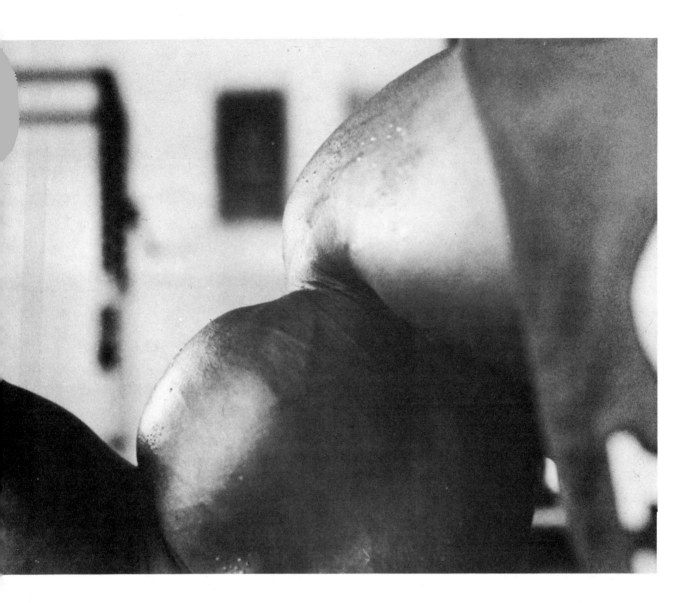

## Going for It

This is as far as I can take you in learning the freestyle way to train naturally for bodybuilding results. You *will* succeed if you want it badly enough. Just train consistently hard and don't miss workouts unless you are actually too physically ill to train.

It's difficult in a book like this to answer all of your potential questions. So if you don't understand something, need a more advanced program, or just want to comment on something, feel free to contact me:

Bill Reynolds
Editor in Chief, *Flex*
21100 Erwin Street
Woodland Hills, CA 91367

I'll write back as quickly as my schedule permits. Pump iron!

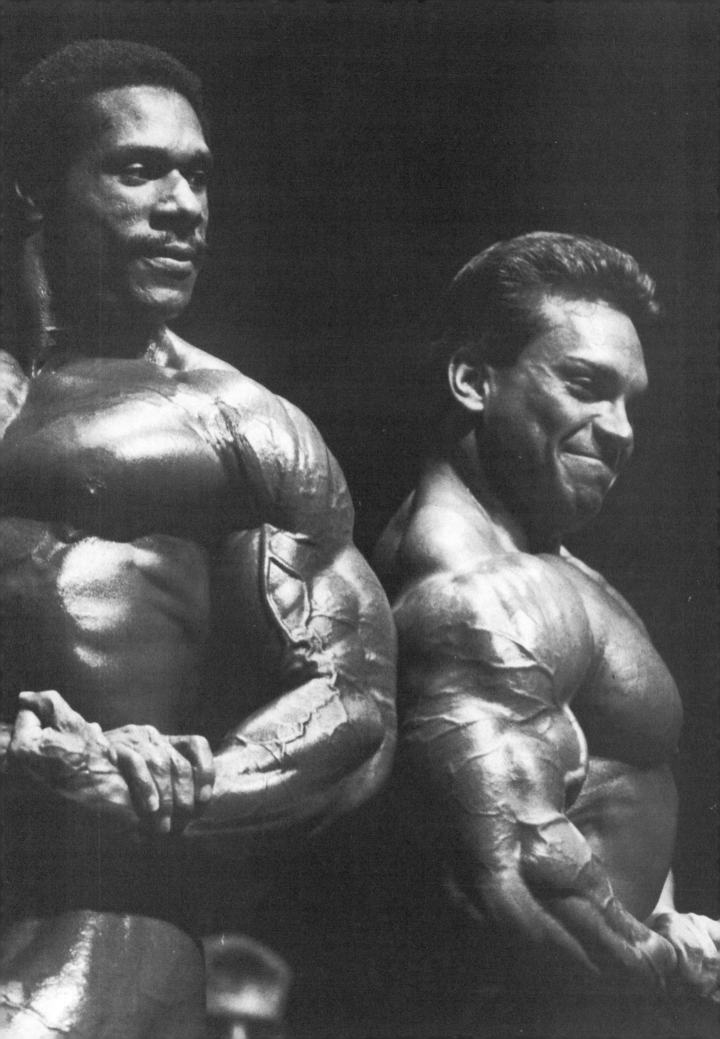

# Suggested Readings

In addition to my own books (listed at the beginning of this mental training manual), I recommend the following texts.

Durkheim, Karfried Graf. *Zen and Us.* New York: Dutton, 1982.

Garfield, Charles, Ph.D., and Bennett, Hal Z. *Peak Performance.* Los Angeles: Tarcher, 1984.

Herrigel, Eugen. *Zen in the Art of Archery.* New York: Pantheon, 1953.

Hyams, Joe. *Zen in the Martial Arts.* Los Angeles: Tarcher, 1979.

Leonard, George. *The Ultimate Athlete.* New York: Viking, 1975.

◀ Mike Christian and Rich Gaspari battle for the elusive title of IFBB Mr. Olympia.

McDonald, Kathleen. *How to Meditate—A Practical Guide.* London: Wisdom Publications, 1984.

Persig, Robert M. *Zen and the Art of Motorcycle Maintenance.* New York: Quill, 1974.

Ross, Nancy Wilson, ed. *The World of Zen.* New York: Vintage Books, 1960.

Suzuki, Daisetz T. *Zen and Japanese Culture.* Princeton, NJ: Princeton-Bollingen, 1973.

——. *The Awakening of Zen.* Boston: Shambhala, 1980.

Tutko, Thomas. *Sports Psyching.* Los Angeles, Tarcher, 1976.

Watts, Alan W. *The Way of Zen.* New York: Viking, 1975.